Natural Animal Healing

An Earth Lodge Pocket Guide to Holistic Pet Wellness

By Maya Cointreau

An Earth Lodge® Publication
Roxbury, Connecticut

*** This book contains valuable information carefully researched, but it is not intended to take the place of proper veterinary care and expertise. Please seek qualified professional care for health problems. ***

All Text & Artwork Copyright 2006, 2009 & 2015, Maya Cointreau

All rights reserved, including the right to reproduce this work in any form whatsoever, without written permission, except in the case of brief quotation in critical articles or reviews. All information in this Earth Lodge® book is based on the experiences of the author. For information contact Earth Lodge®, 12 Church St., Roxbury, CT 06783 or visit Earth Lodge® online at earthlodgebooks.com

Printed & Published in the U.S.A.
by Earth Lodge®
ISBN 978-1-944396-01-5

Earth Lodge® is a registered trademark.

Also by Maya Cointreau:

Practical Reiki Symbol Primer

The Comprehensive Vibrational Healing Guide

The Healing Properties of Flowers

Grounding and Clearing

The Girls Who Could Series

Equine Herbs & Healing

Natural Animal Healing

The Mudra Book

For Lucas,
and all his brothers and sisters
of the next generation:

May your light shine bright and pure,
inspiring the world to love,
laughter and peace,
as time and time again
you have inspired us.

Table of Contents

Introduction — i

A Bite of History — 1

Barking Up the Right Tree:
Choosing & Using Herbs — 7

Herbs for Pets — 19

Homeopathy & Flower Essences — 112

Essential Oils for your Pet — 135

Support from Mother Earth:
Crystal Healing — 153

Ailments & Their Remedies:
A Table — 161

Pet Communication & Care   175

Bibliography   185

Resources & Supplies

About the Author

> *"If one way be better than another, that you may be sure is nature's way."*~ Aristotle

Introduction

"Healing takes courage, and we all have courage, even if we have to dig a little to find it." ~ Tori Amos

I began this book in 2007 as an herbal for dogs, a follow-up to my last animal healing book, "Equine Herbs & Healing." I opened a new word document, set up a folder that I filled with new research, but little writing got done. Months passed in the fall and through the holidays without a glance at the folder on my desktop loosely labeled "Dog Book." The year ended.

Soon it was January 2008, and I was wrapping up a fulfilling evening of shamanic meditations with a group I lead every month at my store. It came to me that what I needed to write, and what you, dear readers, needed to hear, was a book not merely on canine herbalism, but an introduction to the many alternative therapies available for pets of all kinds these days. This idea was both exciting and daunting.

Could I really write such a book? Could so much information really be contained within one cover?

My inner voice and spirit guides all firmly responded "YES!" I ruminated on the project for another month, returning to it just before February.

Here is where you find me today: writing the beginning of a new book which I hope will serve as an enjoyable introduction to natural healing for your pets, and also as a springboard into further research on healing in general. Do not take my word on these therapies as final. Read other books. Go on the Internet. Contact holistic vets and healers in your area. Use your intuition, and listen to your inner voice.

There are vast resources of information and knowledge available on this planet at this time. Do not hesitate to use them. This book is designed to give you a basic knowledge of alternative holistic healing modalities that are available to you as a pet owner.

I do not believe that the knowledge of healing is a privilege: it is your birthright. You can heal yourself. You can heal your pets. Only you can decide, and *know*, what is going to be the most appropriate form of therapy for your family or your pet.

This book is in no way meant to dismiss or supplant veterinary and pharmaceutical treatment and knowledge. I believe that science has many wonderful lessons to show us, just as I believe that the therapies discussed in this book have much to offer. Veterinary diagnosis is an invaluable tool, and often presents the first step towards healing in many cases. My own veterinarian, Dr. Paul Elwell, is a compassionate godsend who has helped my family and friends with innumerable pet illnesses, made house calls when he was supposed to be fishing just to check in on newly whelped puppies, and helped us bring more than one animal back from the brink of death.

I hope you will enjoy this book and that it will help you as you walk through life with your beloved animal companions.

Let the healing begin!

The Author
January 30, 2009

"The art of healing comes from nature, not from the physician. Therefore the physician must start from nature, with an open mind." ~
Philipus Aureolus Paracels

CHAPTER ONE

A Bite of History

"Healing," Papa would tell me, "is not a science, but the intuitive art of wooing nature."
~ W. H. Auden

Every culture has its own tradition of healing: herbs and plants that have been prized for centuries or millennia for their healing properties, revered stones or talismans used by priests to ward off disease, legends of sacred waters, juices or muds. Archaeologists have found herbal documents from Egypt dating from 3000 BCE, and acupuncture tools designed to influence the flow of energy, or Chi, in the body have been found in China dating from 8000 BCE. The first human crops consisted of over two hundred different plants, many of which were grown for their medicinal qualities.

Today, a vast number of medicines still derive from an original plant form. The World Health Organization reports that at least a quarter of Western medicine derives from plants, and that the modern uses of almost three quarters of those medicines are [the same as] the traditional herbal treatments.

With the modern sentiment that animals are not beneath man, but interconnected and to be protected, so has their medical treatment progressed to the point where we have animal communicators, massage therapists, and herbalists who are willing to take a closer look at animals as sentient beings with knowledge to share.

Many species of animals have been documented self-medicating with herbs. Wild chimpanzees will seek out medicinal herbs to ingest when they are ill, plants which they do not normally eat. Horses will seek out the appropriate herbs for their condition when they are lucky to live in a pasture that has herbs in addition to the usual well-groomed forage grass. In China, there is an old folk-tale of how a farmer discovered the valued herb, San Qi, when he watched a snake heal itself by eating this "weed." German scientists have documented injured otters, fish and dolphins rolling in sea algae in the Sargasso Sea to tend to their wounds.

By watching animals closely and listening more intently to their communication, whether it is through body language, purring, or an animal communicator, we can heal animals more effectively. Animal scientist Dr. Temple Grandin has been able to improve livestock handling facility conditions immensely nationwide by providing new insight to how cattle and other animals destined for consumption feel as they enter slaughterhouses and other facilties. Through her own intuition and sensitivities Dr. Grandin has been able to determine how things which most humans would overlook, such as stray shadows, will induce panic in cattle, and applics her observations to make animals' final hours calmer and less fearful, simultaneously making it a smoother process for the humans involved in livestock transport and handling.

Now, many people are delving even deeper into the realm of animal understanding through animal communication. Animal communication is the name for the simple, often wordless, communication a human can have with another animal. Sonya Fitzpatrick has brought animal communication to the masses through television on her show "The Pet Psychic," much as John Edwards has done for mediumship. Only a decade ago, such animal communicators worked primarily helping clients diagnose their pet's medical issues and remedy "inappropriate" behavior: Now, many of them are trying to spread the word, and share their gift with the rest of the world in a more enriching way. Workshops, books and CDs have sprouted up throughout the world to help the common man speak with animals. An open heart and a willing mind seem to be all you need to succeed.

While the idea of hands on healing has been around for millennia and the transcendentalists and rosicrucians of the 19th century discussed many "new age" ideas, it was during the last half of the twentieth century that we saw a surge in the development of alternative healing therapies. Dr. Mikao Usui of Yago, Japan developed Reiki on Mt. Kurama in 1914 and it spread rapidly throughout the west after the initiations of 22 Reiki Masters by Mrs. Hawayo Takata between 1970 and 1980; Barabara Brennan, a former NASA physicist, wrote "Hands of Light: A Guide to Healing Through the Human Energy Field" in 1989 which was a Bantam New Age bestseller and further fueled mainstream interest in hands-on energy healing techniques. Countless books were written on chakras, energy healing, chi, yoga and more: in the beginning most were met with ridicule or ignored, but with the backing of stars like the Beatles, Sting and Jacksons, such unusual ideas have slowly infiltrated mainstream thinking. A large percentage of nurses in the medical community are Reiki certified, and Yoga has become as popular in United States as football. The world is shifting.

Quantum physicists are proving that

the world will shift to meet our expectations. **Expect healing. Expect miracles.** Expectation, coupled with knowledge, results in a better, healed reality. This is the first step to a healthy pet, home, and heart.

CHAPTER TWO

Barking Up the Right Tree: Choosing and Using Remedies

"Science must begin with myths."
~ Sir Karl Popper

There are thousands of plants on this planet, and they all have various medicinal or nutritional properties. Some are very mild, working to gently cool or heat the body, while others stimulate the heart or help the liver regenerate. Every culture has its own pharmacopoeia of herbs, just as every herbalist has his or her own favorite arsenal of herbs that they use most often. Where some use dandelion as a blood cleanser, others prefer burdock. In this book we will be concerning ourselves primarily with herbs from the European and Native American traditions. There are already many wonderful books on Chinese herbs, which also have great value in veterinary applications.

When choosing herbs for your pet, I always suggest looking on the internet to see if there are any new scientific studies about the herb and its effect on that species. New studies and data are being presented every month, due to increased interest being generated in herbs in recent years.

Many herbs work similarly in most species, but one must always take each species' specialized mechanics into consideration. Cats have much faster metabolisms and sensitive nervous systems than dogs, horses or humans. Herbs like Valerian and St. John's Wort that affect the nervous system should be avoided, as they may cause seizures in some cats.

Preparing Herbs

The most natural way to use herbs is of of course in their natural form, dried or fresh, mixed with food or fed straight from the hand. This method works very well with horses, cows, goats and other "hay burners." Dogs, cats and rodents are another story entirely. Carnivores and omnivores are more likely to ingest their herbs if they are prepared in their food or water. Indeed, their digestive systems are not designed to extract nutrients as efficiently from plants, and they will enjoy greater benefits if the herbs are already broken down for them.

Herbs can be used internally and externally in a variety of ways. Different animals and situations call for different applications. This chapter will teach you when and how to make these herbal remedies, and more.

INFUSIONS:

Herbal infusions are made the same way as a cup of tea, except the herbs are allowed to steep longer in the water, creating a flavorful water that has been gently infused with all the medicinal and nutritional qualities of an herb. They can be used in a variety of ways. Infusions can be added to animal drinking water for a mild effect, or tube-fed to weakened, dehydrated animals. You can use them to cleanse wounds, or as part of your pet's bathing routine. A rosemary infusion used as a rinse will make your pet's coat shine and soothe tired muscles, while chamomile will bring out blonde and lighter highlights. Soak a cloth in yarrow and calendula and hold it against the skin to draw out infections.

To make an herbal infusion, bring water to a boil in a steel or glass pot, and then remove from the heat. (Aluminum and copper are both reactive metals and should not be used to prepare herbal solutions.) Add one tablespoon of dried herbs, or three tablespoons of fresh herbs, per cup of hot water. Cover and let steep for 13 - 15 minutes. (The longer it steeps, the stronger it will be. Dried roots should steep a bit longer, 20 - 30 minutes.) Strain the liquid before use through a cheesecloth or fine metal strainer. Let cool and use, or place in an airtight container to store in the refrigerator for 3 - 5 days.

BRACES:

A brace is a strong, invigorating liquid solution that is used on soaked bandages to treat a sprain or minor wound. Braces are also used to wash down horses after hard rides to soothe the entire body. Braces can be made out of very strong infusions (steeped for 20 –30 minutes in a non-aluminum pot) or by adding a teaspoon of herbal extracts to a cup of water and cup of vegetable glycerin (to wash an animal down) or to a cup of witch hazel and a cup of distilled water (to treat a wound). Once you have prepared the brace solution, soak bandages or cotton clothes in the liquid, and apply to the wound for 20 – 60 minutes, securing with additional dressings as needed.

POULTICES:

Poultices are used similarly to braces, by placing them directly on wounds to draw out infections and bring down swelling. Poultices can be made with fresh or dried herbs. First, place your herbs in a heat-resistant glass, ceramic or steel bowl. Next, bring a pot of water to a full boil (for open wound treatments, boil the water for a minimum of 15 minutes to kill any bacteria in the water, or use distilled water), and pour a small amount of the hot water over the herbs, soaking them until they are softened. Strain the herbs, saving the infused liquid as a brace for later treatment or to add to the animal's drinking water, depending on what herbs you are using. When the softened herbs reach body-temperature, they are safe to put directly on the affected area. Secure a sterile cloth bandage to keep the poultice in place.

A wonderful example of an herbal poultice is yarrow, which will stop bleeding, clean the wound and speed healing. The infused water can also be added to your horse's drinking water to help heal the wound from the inside out.

Calendula is a good herb to poultice on hot spots to soothe the damage skin and reduce irritation.

TINCTURES:

Herbal tinctures are cold infusions of herbs that generally take two – six weeks to steep. They are one of the easiest ways to give herbs to small domestic animals in the home: simply add a few drops to your pet's drinking water or food. Some herbs, such as Dandelion and Nettle, are beneficial for all pets, and can be used in a communal water bowl.

Instead of being infused in water, tinctures are made in high-proof alcohol such as brandy or vodka, vinegar or vegetable glycerin. To treat animals, I recommend using apple cider vinegar, which is good for their digestive systems and is much more palatable.

Tinctures properly stored in air-tight, glass containers can be stored for 18 – 36 months. Wide-mouthed glass jars with plastic or glass lids work best: glass jars with metal lids are not recommended, as the metal can react with vinegar and corrode. Although tinctures take time to prepare initially, in the long run they are much easier to use: in an emergency, the herbs are ready to use, with waiting time. Keep a few choice herbs tinctured and at the ready, such as Yarrow for accidents involving bleeding and Cat's Claw or Boneset for bacterial infections.

To prepare a tincture, fill the jar halfway with chopped, dried herbs (fresh herbs contain water and can lead to spoilage) and top with vinegar. Close the jar and store in a cool, dark place for two to six weeks. The longer it infuses, the stronger the tincture will be. Woody stems and roots should be infused for the full six weeks in order to be sure you have extracted their full potency. When the tincture is ready, strain off the liquid, remove the herbs, and return the liquid to the jar. Store in a cool, dark place for up to 36 months. 15-30 drops of a tincture is considered equivalent to one cup of a fresh herbal infusion, depending on the strength of your infusion.

POWDERED HERBS:

These days, you can find standardized, powdered herbs in capsules at most pharmacies and health food stores. These powdered herbs offer another convenient way to give herbs to smaller pets. Choose a reputable brand, such as Nature's Way or Nature's Herbs, and then simply open the capsule and sprinkle the powder over your pet food. Stir, and feed. Generally, a half-capsule is plenty for one cat, or one-three capsules for a dog depending on size.

INFUSED OILS:

Infused oils can be used directly on skin or added to custom salves or balms.

First, you begin with a carrier oil. For animals I recommend using olive or grapeseed oil. Sweet almond and apricot oils both contain trace amounts of cyanide and should not be used on animals which groom themselves. There are several ways to infuse carrier oils. Either fresh or dried herbs may be used, although we prefer to use dried herbs because the water content of fresh herbs may lead to spoilage. If you do use fresh herbs, always make sure that they are washed clean and fully dried off before you infuse them.

The fastest way to infuse an oil is by heating the oil and herbs over the lowest heat on your stove for twenty minutes. The warmth allows the herbal properties to seep into the oil quite quickly, making this an efficient method. However, heat also accelerates the breakdown process of oils, which will shorten their shelf life. When using this method, be sure you are use grapeseed or coconut oil. You can also use the heat of the sun to infuse oils, by placing a jar filled with the herbs and the oil in a sunny window for several days. Olive oil is not suitable for heat infusion if you are planning on storing it for more than a week, although the life of any infused oil can be prolonged by adding one-half teaspoon of vitamin E or 5 drops of benzoin essential oil per cup of carrier oil.

Cold-infusion poses the least amount of stress to your carrier oil, and is easy to perform. Again, simply place the herbs is a glass jar, cover, and place in a dark cupboard at room temperature for 2-6 weeks. When the herbal infusion has reached the strength you desire, strain and store. An oil prepared by cold infusion will last for 6 to 18 months.

SALVES:

A salve, or balm, is a wax and oil based ointment that is great for wound treatments and skin conditioning. Solid and long-lasting, a salve is a convenient way to take herbal remedies on the road. In medieval times, wives would often make up a salve for their husbands to take into battle or on long voyages.

Salves are easy to make. You can use fresh or dried herbs, or essential oils, or all three in your salves. The simplest way to make a salve is to heat one part shaved beeswax in four parts carrier oil on the stove or in a microwave, just enough to melt the beeswax. The wax will melt best if you cut it into small pieces or use beeswax beads.

Remove the mixture from the heat and stir it a few times. If you are using an herbal cold-infused carrier oil, then your job is done. If you are adding essential oils to the mixture, add them now and stir again. Pour the mixture into a suitable non-reactive container and let cool. It will harden as it cools, and store for 12-18 months, depending on what kind of oils you use. Adding a drop of benzoin essential oil or the oil from a 400 IU vitamin E oil capsule for every 4 ounces of salve will also prolong your salve's shelf life.

CHAPTER THREE

Herbs for Animals

"The only work that will ultimately bring any good to any of us is the work of contributing to the healing of the world." ~ *Marianne Williamson*

This chapter will introduce you to a myriad of herbs and their general properties, as well as species specific guidelines or restrictions. Not all herbs are good for all species, and research should always be done before administering herbs to see if any new scientific data has come forth regarding effects or dosage information.

Many herbs have not been tested to determine their safety during pregnancy for any animals, including humans. For this reason, most herbs should be avoided during pregnancy, and often lactation, unless they are specifically noted as safe. Herbs which are definitively known to induce labor or defects are also noted.

General Dosage Guidelines

Dosages vary from species to species, by weight, and depending on how you are administering the herbs. Of course, dosages can change depending on the strength of an herb or extract. Compare extracts to each other: if the dosage is much smaller compared to other brands, cut the recommended dosages given below in half. If your pet is picky, start off with smaller doses so that it can get used to the taste.

Herbs can be given daily as tinctures added to pet water or food; as dried, cut or ground herbs sprinkled on top of food; cooked with rice (dogs especially love this); or as infusions, added to drinking water. For acute conditions, try giving herbs twice daily, once in the evening and once at night.

Cats

Tinctures: *5 to 10 drops of tincture in water or mixed with food per day.*

Capsules: *½ to 1 capsule of powdered herb, opened and mixed with food per day.*

Dogs

Tinctures: *Small Dogs (5-30 lbs): 5 to 15 drops of tincture in water or mixed with food per day. Medium Dogs (30-80 lbs) 15 to 30 drops of tincture in water or mixed with food per day. Large Dogs (80 lbs and over) 30 to 45 drops of tincture in water or mixed with food per day.*

Capsules: *Small Dogs: ½ to 1 capsule of powdered herb, opened and mixed with food per day or fed directly to dog. Medium Dogs: 1 – 2 capsule. Large Dogs: 2 –3 capsules.*

Dried Herbs in Rice: Cook the herbs and rice together, 1 tbs dried herbs or 1 tsp fresh herbs per cup of dried rice. Small Dogs: ¼ to ½ cup cooked rice. Medium Dogs: ½ to 1 cup cooked rice. Large Dogs: 1 to 1 ½ cup cooked rice.

Infusion: Small Dogs: 1/8 to ¼ cup infusion. Medium Dogs: ¼ to ½ cup infusion. Large Dogs: ½ to 1 cup infusion.

Horses

Tinctures: *Small Horses (up to 5 hands): 15 to 30 drops of tincture in water or mixed with feed per day. Medium Horses (5-6 ½ hands): 30 to 60 drops of tincture Large Horses (6 ½ hands and greater) 60 to 90 drops of tincture.*

Capsules: *Small Horses: 2 to 3 capsules of powdered herb, opened and mixed with feed per day or administered directly. Medium Horses: 3 to 4 capsules. Large Horses: 4 to 5 capsules*

Dried & Fresh Herbs: Small Horses: 1 to 3 tsp dried and cut herbs per day with feed. Medium Horses: 1 to 2 tbs dried and cut herbs. Large Horses: 2 to 3 tbs dried and cut herbs. Dried herbs are more potent than fresh herbs,: for fresh herbs, use twice the dosage.

Infusion: Small Horses: 1 cup of infusion added to drinking water. Medium Horses: 2 cups of infusion. Large Horses: 3 cups of infusion.

Note: Always test your herbs for palatability, especially when adding them to your horse's drinking water. Many horses love the flavor of apple cider vinegar, which can be added to the water (1 -2 cups per 5 gallon bucket) to make herbs more palatable and to aid your horse's digestion. For goats, sheep and miniature breeds, cut the dosages for small horses in half.

Next, you will find a glossary of herbal terms which are commonly used by herbalists to describe medicinal properties.

Herbal Properties Glossary

Adaptogen: adapts its effect to what the body needs

Alterative: increases overall health & tissue renewal

Analgesic: pain reliever

Anodyne: pain reliever

Antacid: reduces acidity in stomach & gut

Anthelmintic: expels worms & parasites

Antibiotic: kills infections

Antifungal: kills fungal infections

Anti-inflammatory: reduces inflammation in & on the body

Antimicrobial: destroys micro-organisms; i.e. bacteria & fungi

Antiseptic: inhibits growth of bacteria & other infections

Antispasmodic: relieves spasms

Antitussive: relieves coughs

Aperient: gently moves the bowels; gentle laxative

Astringent: draws and binds together soft organic tissues

Aromatic: distinctive fragrant smell

Antiemetic: discourages vomiting

Antioxidant: scavenges free radicals to limit cellular damage

Antirheumatic: relieves arthritis

Antiseptic: cleans wounds and discourages infection by preventing the growth of bacteria

Calmative: sedative & calming

Carminative: helps expel gas to relieve cramps and colic

Demulcent: soothes inflammation

Detoxification: eliminates impurities from the blood & supports the liver

Diaphoretic: increases perspiration

Diuretic: increases and encourages the flow of urine

Electrolytes: natural body salts: sodium bicarbonate, sodium chloride, and potassium chloride

Emetic: causes vomiting

Emmenagogue: promotes menstruation, abortive

Emollient: softens the skin or mucous membranes

Expectorant: expels mucus from the respiratory tract

Febrifuge: reduces fever

Flavonoids: plant constituents that affect healing

Galactagogue: increases the production of milk

Hepatic: drains and cleanses the liver

Hypertensive: raises blood pressure

Hypotensive: lowers blood pressure

Immuno-stimulant: stimulates & supports the immune system

Laxative: relieves constipation by promoting bowel movement

Mucilage: demulcent that soothes mucous membranes

Nervine: affects the nervous system

Nutritive: of nutritional or nourishing value

Phytotherapy: therapeutic plant remedies in medicines.

Refrigerant: cools; relieves fever or heat

Sedative: calms and relaxes, soothing nervous tension

Stimulant: energy producing

Stomachic: aids digestion

Styptic: controls bleeding

Tonic: cleanses and promotes healthy bodily functions

Uterine Stimulant: promotes uterine contractions

Vermifuge: expels worms

Volatile Oils: plant oils easily vaporized with heat or pressure

Vulnerary: heals wounds

Herbs & Their Properties

Astragalus

Astragalus membranaceus, Astragalus mongholicus

Parts Used: roots

Properties: alterative, anti-bacterial, anti-inflammatory, diaphoretic, diuretic, immuno-stimulant, stimulant.

Astragalus is very instrumental in augmenting flagging immune systems, and boosting overall health. In Chinese traditional medicine (TCM) it is generally combined with other strengthening herbs, being used historically to raise energy levels, treat chronic diseases and cancers, and significantly improve liver, kidney and adrenal function. It has been shown in recent scientific studies to have beneficial effects on heart functions, and to possibly improve chemotherapy benefits, and more studies are currently targeting astragalus as a cancer adjunct therapy.

Astragalus is so good at raising immune responses that when it is used against infections it can increase or prolong fevers. Therefore, I generally do not use it if there is already a fever present, and if a fever presents while using astragalus, I recommend backing off of it for several days. Once the fever presents, the immune system is already doing its job!

Because it hones the immune system, without actually over-stimulating it as Echinacea can sometimes do, astragalus has been used traditionally to help treat those with multiple allergies, where the cause is believed to be a faulty immune system: Astragalus has the ability to "reboot" the immune system, similar to Cat's Claw.

Astragalus can lower blood pressure and blood sugar, so if your pet is already on diabetic medications or has very low blood pressure, Astragalus is not indicated. Due to the sensitivity of feline metabolisms, cut feline dosages in half when using astragalus.

Barberry

Berberis vulgaris

Parts Used: berries, roots, bark

Properties: antibacterial, antimicrobial, anti-inflammatory, astringent, demulcent, febrifuge, hypotensive, immuno-stimulant, sedative, uterine stimulant.

Barberry was used by the Egyptians for thousands of years, and is still widely used today in Iran to treat gallbladder and digestive disorders. Barberry's name actually derives from its prolific use in England were it can be found throughout the land forming impervious hedges which bar all trespassers. While it is generally safe for occasional livestock consumption, its long thorns make it unlikely forage in the pasture, making it a very good natural fence for horses.

Barberry contains notable quantities of the antibacterial alkaloids berberine and berbamine. It increases white blood cell production and is often used to treat diarrhea, intestinal parasites, and viral, bacterial and fungal infections. For kidney or bladder stones, barberry can be very effective given in half-doses three times a day.

Note: Barberry is contraindicated in pregnant or lactating animals, and in animals with decreased liver function.

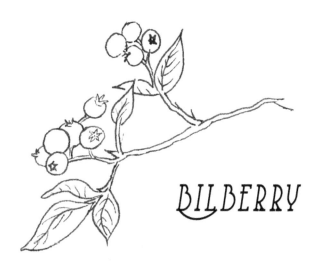

Bilberry

Accinium myrtillus

Parts Used: berries and leaves

Properties: astringent, antibacterial, antioxidant, antiseptic, laxative, diuretic, refrigerant.

Bilberry has a long tradition as an eye treatment in Europe, even having been used during World War II in Britain to improve airplane pilots' night vision.

Taken internally, bilberry can lower blood pressure behind the eyes and deliver more oxygen to the eyes, and are an herbal remedy for macular degeneration, glaucoma and cataracts. This is attributed in large part to the fact that bilberries contain *anthocyanidins* and *proanthocyanidins*, anti-oxidants that can reduce inflammation, strengthen blood vessels and regulate proper blood flow throughout the body.

Bilberry leaves, like its "cousin" blueberry, are native to North America, and have valuable astringent qualities as a diuretic and to treat urinary tract issues, diarrhea and colic. They can help prevent bladder or kidney stones, and benefit a variety of digestive conditions. Due to their anti-oxidant properties, bilberries are also believed to be beneficial in adjunct cancer therapies. Bilberry allows wounds and tissues to heal more effectively, and Native Americans traditionally washed external wounds with bilberry infusions to speed healing.

Bloodroot

Sanguinaria Canadensis

Parts Used:

Properties: alterative, emetic, experctorant, tonic

Bloodroot has been used extensively in many native and herbal traditions to treat external cancers, tumors and warts. It is noted for its ability to encourage mutated cells to self-destruct, while not affecting healthy skin tissue. Recently, bloodroot has been steadily declining in the wild and should not be wild-crafted. Seek bloodroot through reputable sources who have taken care to ensure the proliferation of this fragile and beautiful plant.

Bloodroot is toxic when administered internally, and extreme caution should always be taken that animals can not lick it off their bodies. Bot fly larvae on horses can be killed by careful application of bloodroot. In general, Goldenseal has many of the same anti-growth properties as bloodroot, with gentler effects. Because it is gentler, it also works more slowly.

Note: Bloodroot is toxic to the nervous system when ingested, particularly to cats. Use only when supervised by a qualified practitioner.

Boneset

Eupatorium perfoliatum,

Parts Used: leaves and new blossoms

Properties: aperient, antispasmodic, diaphoretic, emetic, febrifuge, stimulant, tonic.

After being properly dried, boneset acts as a tonic and febrifuge, strengthening weakened constitutions and combating recurring fevers.

European research has found that boneset's capacity to stimulate the immune system and combat bacterial infections make boneset a powerful instrument for occasional use. It was used extensively throughout the United States by Native Americans and settlers alike, combating influenza and common colds.

Its name derives from its treatment of "breakbone fever," or dengue fever, which is generally accompanied by joint pain. Boneset is quite adept at alleviating, along with pains in the bones. Ancient herbalists used to see an herb's appearance as an indicator of its properties: boneset's leaves actually appear skewered by its stem. Given to horses that have been badly bruised or suffered bone and ligament injuries, boneset may lessen their discomfort.

When taken warm, boneset encourages the passing of fecal matter, and can be used in this manner to help relieve an impacted animal.

Note: Boneset taken in large doses can cause diarrhea. Only use boneset after it has been dried to eliminate the presence of tremerol, a toxic chemical. Also, related species of Eupatorium have been found to contain pyrolizzidine alkaloids. Phytochemical research has yet to conclude whether or not Boneset also contains these alkaloids, however, there is concern that boneset taken over long-term periods may lead to liver damage if it does them contain . Therefore, use boneset only in small, short-term bursts, and always in conjunction with milk thistle to counteract possible side-effects.

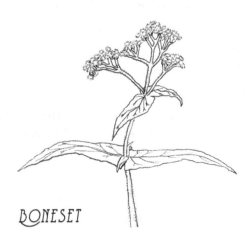

BONESET

Borage

Borago Officinalis

Parts Used: leaves and oil.

Properties: anti-inflammatory, aperient, diaphoretic, diuretic, demulcent, emollient, febrifuge, galactogogue, refrigerant, stimulant.

Borage is a very soothing mucilaginous herb, both inside and outside the body with mild anti-inflammatory properties. It can be used internally to treat fevers and clear respiratory congestion, as well as to soothe and restore stressed adrenal glands. The ancient Romans used it as a mild stimulant, and it has been used throughout the ages as an herbal remedy for depressed spirits.

Borage oil is particularly rich in GLA (gamma linoleni acid) and fights plaque deposits in arteries, as well as delivering a potent punch to allergies and skin conditions. Borage seeds contain trace amounts of pyrolizzidine alkaloids which can be damaging to the liver, but scientific studies done on the oil derived from the seeds have determined that the alkaloids are not present in the oil. Commercially-prepared borage oil and borage leaves are both generally believed to be safe and PA free. Externally, borage is extremely useful in reducing bruises and inflamed muscles or joints.

Note: Borage can over-stimulate the nervous system in large doses; Cut dosages in half for felines. It is not recommended for pregnant or nursing animals for the same reason.

BURDOCK

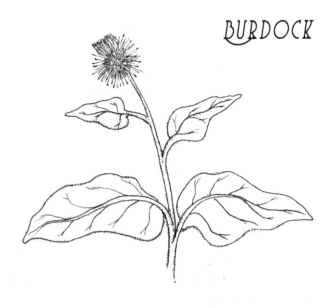

Burdock

Arctium lappa, Arctium minus

Parts Used: leaves and roots

Properties: alterative, demulcent, diaphoretic, diuretic, nutritive.

Burdock is a wonderful blood-cleansing herb that detoxifies the liver, blood, kidneys and entire lymphatic system. In China, it has long been used as the foremost detox herb, and to treat arthritis. In Western herbal medicine, it has a long history of being used to reduce inflammation in joints and muscles, and help lower fevers. Lesser Burdock (*arctium minus*) can be used similarly.

Burdock can be used to treat eye infections by removing unwanted substances from the body and healing irritated tissue. Burdock is part of many herbal anti-cancer regimens due to its ability to remove environmental toxins from the body and encourage healthy bone marrow. It is a very gentle, safe herb to use long-term for such detoxifying purposes.

Used externally, burdock root benefits many skin conditions, from rashes and sores, to burns and minor wounds. Infused in oil and applied directly to the skin, burdock also has a reputation for its ability to re-grow and strengthen hair. Leaf poultices relieve skin irritations, sores, and tumors, and have good antiseptic properties. It has not been tested on pregnant and nursing animals, and internal use should generally be avoided in such conditions.

Calendula

Calendula officinalis

Parts Used: flower petals

Properties: antispasmodic, anti-inflammatory, antiseptic, detoxifying, mildly estrogenic, astringent, diaphoretic, stimulant, vulnerary.

Calendula, or Pot Marigold, is one of the most versatile herbs in Western herbalism; these vibrant orange blossoms, whether fresh or dried, have significant antiseptic and healing qualities. Internally, calendula stimulates circulation while cleansing the liver and blood, making it very useful in the treatment of bruises and sprains.

Calendula provides soothing treatment for flea bites, burns, systemic skin disorders such as eczema, and fungal conditions like ringworm and thrush. Nothing surpasses calendula in its ability to heal and cleanse the skin when used as a external wash or taken internally to heal from the inside out.

Cat's Claw

Uncaria tomentosa

Parts Used: bark

Properties: abortive, anti-inflammatory, antioxidant, anti-rheumatic, antiviral, immuno-stimulant, kidney tonic.

Cat's Claw, or Una de Gato, is a long, thorny vine from the Amazon that is gaining popularity throughout the west as a potent immuno-stimulant and urinary tonic. The Ashaninka Indians of Peru use it not only to heal the body, but to strengthen the spiritual aspect of those who take it. Cat's claw works on the immune system by strengthening white blood cell performance. Many believe cat's claw also helps memory function and may combat Alzheimers: The National Institute for Aging is currently researching this aspect of cat's claw.

Cat's claw can be useful in treating chronic inflammatory conditions of the bowels, kidneys and bladder, especially when they stemmed originally from a bacterial infection. Similarly, early studies indicate that cat's claw may have positive effects on viral and parasitic infections such as Feline Leukemia Virus and Lymes Disease when used in conjunction with conventional therapies.

Note: Cat's claw has been used for centuries to prevent pregnancies in the Amazon, and is not safe for use with pregnant animals.

Celery

Apium graveolens

Parts Used: seeds, stems, & leaves

Properties: antirheumatic, anti-inflammatory, antispasmodic, carminative, diuretic, emmenagogue, nervine, stimulant, stomachic, tonic.

In Ancient Egypt, celery was used as a tonic to relieve swelling in joints and muscles, to soothe stomachaches and to cure headaches. It has been cultivated for more than 3000 years in China and the Middle East due to its cleansing, tonifying effect on the entire body. Celery can be added to homemade dog and cat food to help cleanse their bodies and promote healthy digestion. Celery juice, especially when mixed with organic carrot juice, strengthens debilitated bodies after prolonged illness.

Medicinally, celery seeds are generally the part of the plant that herbalists use. Today, celery seeds are used primarily to promote regular urination, which can benefit nerves, arthritis, lung and respiratory ailments, fevers and liver problems. They also help regulate and lower blood sugar levels and blood pressure. Celery seeds are also a mild sedative, and can tantalize some cats the way catnip does.

Note: Not for use with pregnant animals.

CHAMOMILE

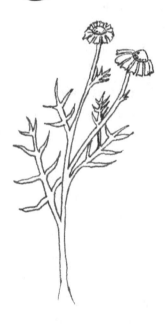

Chamomile

Matricaria chamomilla, Chamemelum nobile

Parts Used: flowers & leaves

Properties: anodyne, anti-inflammatory, antiallergenic, antispasmodic, carminative, diaphoretic, emmenagogue, galactagogue, nervine, tonic, sedative, stomachic, vulnerary.

Chamomile has long been known for its relaxing, soothing properties. It is used throughout western civilization to calm nerves, promote sleep and help relieve indigestion, colic and headaches. It combines extremely well with other herbs to benefit all illnesses that derive or suffer from stress: general pain and inflammation remedies will benefit from the inclusion of chamomile, which is calming and relaxing to the muscles, nerves and joints in problem areas.

This versatile herb is a fine insecticide, can relieve eyestrain when used as a wash, and is valuable to treat hay fever and asthma; an external skin application helps relieve eczema and itchy skin patches, especially when used in conjunction with calendula. Similarly, skin and respiratory allergies can benefit from small doses of chamomile, which will relieve the stress induced by allergies.

Chamomile will also help relieve muscle cramps during menstruation and after given birth, and it increases milk production in mammals. Not only is it a safe herb to give nursing mothers, it calms babies and reduces teething pain and irritability. A cup of the infusion added daily to your puppy's drinking water when it is getting its adult teeth (from between 4-8 months old) may very well save your shoes, pillows, books and other precious items from destruction at this age.

Note: Chamomile should not be given to pregnant animals as it may help induce early labor.

Chaste Tree

Vitex agnus-castus

Parts Used: berry

Properties: adaptogen, anti-galactogogue, emmenagogue, vulnerary.

While Chaste tree berry contains no hormonal compounds, it contains flavonoids which work similarly to the hormone progesterone to stimulate the pituitary gland in the brain. Conversely, it will lower hormones when they are too high. As an adaptogen, it is reputed to regulate female hormone and menstrual cycles, alleviate many symptoms associated with the menstrual cycle such as irritability, muscle pains, and hormonal mood swings. Chaste tree works slowly and gently on the body, and usage generally lasts for 6-12 months, allowing the pituitary function to normalize fully. When used to treat infertility, usage may continue for as long as 24 months. Discontinue usage upon conception.

Chaste tree was traditionally used to stimulate milk production, but studies in rats show that it actually decreases production of the hormone prolactin, so it should not be used while nursing (prolactin is believed to be the primary hormone for stimulating milk production in the mammary glands.) Instead, turn to safe, traditional galactagogues such as chamomile, marshmallow and fenugreek.

Historically, chaste berry was fed to monks to lessen their sexual urges and interest in the female sex. Presumably, this effect stems from the herb's moderating hormonal properties, and may produce similar effects on studs.

Note: Not for use with pregnant or nursing animals.

Cleavers

Galium aparine

Parts Used: leaves, stems

Properties: alterative, aperient, diuretic, refrigerant, tonic.

Internally, cleavers has shown significant benefits to regulating urination and bowel movements, and cleaning all obstructions and infections from the digestive and eliminative tracts with great efficiency. As such, it is particularly recommended for horses forced to experience extra stall-time, whether due to winter conditions, illness or training restrictions. In any case, cleavers, also known as goose grass or bedstraw, will help animals suffering from lack of movement, keeping bodily functions well in tune.

In recent studies, cleavers has been shown to contain anti-inflammatory and anti-tumor properties, as well as showing a propensity for lowering blood pressure.

Cleavers detoxifies the lymphatic system, benefiting allergy and cancer treatments. For the same reason, it is wonderful for animals sensitive to flea bites or mites. Added to drinking water it will help with chronic bladder and kidney stones, while relieving chronic skin conditions and diseases such as eczema and psoriasis. Cleavers is yet another herb that is valuable internally and externally in a variety of therapeutic treatments: salves made from cleavers are soothing to dry, itchy skin rashes.

Clover, Red

Trifolium pratense

Parts Used: flowers

Properties: alterative, anticancer, antispasmodic, antitumor, deobstruant, expectorant, sedative

Red clover is a mild phytoestrogen, and can be used to treat hormonal imbalances. In small, regular doses, red clover will have a calming effect on animals.

A mild herb, red clover helps relieve inflammation and tones the blood, flushing impurities. Similarly, it is an expectorant and can help soothe lung congestion and coughs. American Indians used Red Clover as a salve to treat burns and other skin irritations, and as a poultice to relieve sore eyes. Indeed, European herbalists still use this herb to treat cataracts

A nutritive herb, red clover helps the body assimilate iron and contains a high amount of anti-oxidants, protein and calcium. Historically among herbalists, clover has long been believed to be valuable in the treatment of cancers and ulcers, perhaps because of its anti-oxidant properties.

The National Cancer Institute has more recently confirmed red clover's efficacy as an anti-cancer treatment. To use it as an anti-cancer treatment, red clover may be applied directly to external tumors as a poultice or taken internally as a tea.

Red Clover also improves the soil, as a nitrogen-fixing legume, and is excellent for occasional grazing and fodder for horses as well as a sweet source of nectar for honeybees.

Note: Though generally considered a calming herb, excessive doses may have the opposite effect. Red Clover has been shown to have a contraceptive effect on sheep, and should not be used with breeding animals.

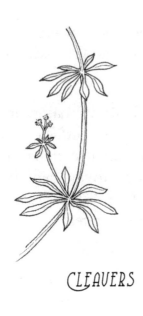

CLEAVERS

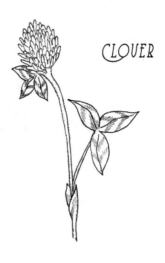

CLOVER

Corn Silk

Zea mayz

Parts used: styles and stigmas of corn (corn silk)

Properties: demulcent, diuretic, hypotensive, urinary tonic

Corn has proved itself to be imminently versatile and nourishing to humans and livestock for thousands of years, so it is no surprise to find that corn silk, the fine hair that we remove from inside the husk when are preparing an ear of corn for dinner, is medicinal. Corn silk is gently relaxes the central nervous system and detoxes the entire body. It is of particular use in urinary and prostate infections, and soothes and relaxes irritated bladders prone to frequent or difficult urination.

For medicinal use, corn silk should always be collected from pesticide-free corn. Its detoxifying action is especially beneficial to the kidneys, and in China it is used primarily to treat jaundice. It reduces fluid retention and can help lower blood pressure, relieving gout and varicose veins.

Corn silk is high in vitamin K and is a wonderful, safe herb to give animals in their last few days of gestation and during birthing to help prevent bleeding problems in both mother and offspring. Externally, corn silk helps heal and sooth wounds and skin irritations.

Dandelion

Taraxacum officinale

Parts Used: leaves and root

Properties: alterative, aperient, astringent, cholagogue, detoxifying, diuretic, galactogogue, lithotriptic, stomachic, tonic.

Dandelion has made its way from its original home in Greece around the entire globe, spreading the message that herbalism really isn't any further than your own back yard. Its Latin name, *Taraxacum officinale*, actually means "official cure of disorders."

Dandelion is a powerful detoxifier and tonic, and is primarily used to cleanse the blood, kidneys and liver as well as the entire digestive tract. Arthritis and rheumatism in animals often stems from improper digestion and blood acidity: dandelion is a natural remedy for all such ailments.

Because of its strong cleansing properties, dandelion will clear many skin rashes and allergies, many of which result from waste and environmental toxins building up in the bloodstream and lymphatic system. For this reason, dandelion is also a good herb to add to any formula designed to combat tumors or cysts. It is reputed to stimulate milk production in nursing animals, and is generally considered safe for all conditions. It can be used during pregnancy to provide many essential vitamins, including calcium and iron, and to alleviate constipation.

Devil's Claw

Harpagophytum radix, & H. procumbens

Parts Used: root

Properties: anodyne, anti-inflammatory, stomachic

Brought to Europe and North America from southern Africa and Madagascar, Devil's Claw has been proven in many scientific studies to reduce inflammation and relieve muscle and joint pain. It is extremely effective when used either internally or externally in the treatment of arthritis and similar chronic conditions, including ligament, tendon, and locomotive disorders. Prolonged usage (six weeks or more) has been shown in studies to improve joint elasticity and mobility. German studies have likened its anti-inflammatory properties to phenylbutazone, or bute, with no toxicity or undesirable side-effects. In fact, it has been shown to improve liver and gall-bladder conditions.

Devil's claw root has also been shown to benefit poor appetites and indigestion. It is considered a uterine stimulant, and should not be used on pregnant or nursing animals.

Echinacea

Echinacea angustifolia, Echinacea purpurea

Parts Used: whole herb

Properties: alterative, antibacterial, antibiotic, antiseptic, antiviral, detoxifying, immune stimulant, vulnerary.

Purple coneflower, or echinacea, is an American native and was used by the Plains Indians as a blood purifier and tonic, as well as to treat toothache and sore throats. In modern herbal medicine, it is primarily used to combat any kind of bacterial or viral infection. It has been shown to increase white blood cell and T-cell production, and raise the body's overall immune system.

Echinacea works well in conjunction with goldenseal for a full-body anti-bacterial cleansing, or with ginseng to stimulate circulation as well. Studies have shown that echinacea is most effective when taken before any contagion is introduced and in the very first stages of infection.

After two weeks, echinacea's effect on the immune system levels off, and most experts agree that it is best to take echinacea for periods of 2-8 weeks, and then 2-4 week period of "rest" when no echinacea is taken, in order for the herb to continue to work to its full effect.

Externally, Native Americans used the root for centuries as an anti-bacterial poultice to treat festering wounds, insect stings and snake bites.

Note: Do not administer to animals with autoimmune disorders or severe allergies.

Elder

Sambucus Canadensis, Sambucus Nigra

Parts Used: dried blue-black berries and white flowers

Properties: anti-inflammatory, antioxidant, antiviral, diuretic, laxative.

American Elder and European Elder may be used interchangeably to treat and ward off viruses and infections. In Europe, the flowers have been studied and used extensively to treat colds, flus and respiratory infections. Native Americans used elder in a similar manner, and also to treat arthritis, and studies on animals have shown elder flower water to have an anti-inflammatory effect. Elderberry is a key ingredient in many herbal immune boosters on the market today, especially for children as elderberries are generally believed to be safe and non-toxic.

Note: The bark and leaves of elderberry contain sambucine, and are both purgative and emetic. They are particularly toxic to cats. Use the dried berries, flowers or extracts only.

ELDER

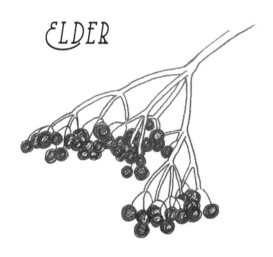

Elecampane

Inula helenium

Parts Used: flower, root

Properties: anti-inflammatory, antimicrobial, antiseptic, astringent, carminative, cholagogue, diaphoretic, diuretic, emmenagogue, expectorant, stimulant, tonic

Also known as horseheal and elfwort, elecampane has a long history in veterinary tradition. It infiltrated European tradition from the East, traveling with the horse-traders of Central Asia. Traditional European herbalists used it to help clear out intestinal worms.

In Ancient Egypt, elecampane was used regularly in cooking to aid digestion. Indeed, elecampane stimulates and clears the digestive tract, reducing phlegm production and working as a general energy tonic.

Its ultimate value is its ability to clear and restore the respiratory and pulmonary systems. In China and Europe today, elecampane is used to clear mucus and benefit asthma and other chronic lung conditions. It is a valuable adjunct when treating kennel cough, especially when combined with thyme and mullein. Due to its ability to increase the intake of oxygen through the lungs, it is also very beneficial for asthma and wheezing cases.

Because of its ability to clear the body of mucus and toxins, elecampane can also be used internally to treat many skin conditions to great effect. In 2005, a study showed that compounds in elecampane have rather potent anti-cancer effects in humans, and it should be considered when researching complementary cancer therapies for pets.

Fenugreek

Trigonella foenum-graecum

Parts Used: seeds

Properties: antidiabetic, galactagogue.

Fenugreek seeds are used throughout the

world to increase milk supply in nursing mothers. Fenugreek seeds have a notable maple syrup taste, making them pleasing to many animals. Studies have shown that it is indeed a very potent galactagogue, capable of increasing supply up to ten-fold. It is also under diverse study as a good anti-diabetic herb, and has been found to increase glucose tolerance in both animals and humans.

Garlic

Allium sativum

Parts Used: bulb

Properties: alterative, antibiotic, antiseptic, antispasmodic, carminative, diaphoretic, digestant, diuretic, expectorant, hypotensive, parasiticide, stimulant.

Native to Asia west of the Himalayas, garlic was considered a deity in Ancient Egypt and was a staple of the Egyptian diet used in a myriad of medicinal remedies: for dog and snake bites, bruises, sore throats, toothaches and infected ears. Cloves of garlic have even been found in the tomb of Tutankhamun.

Garlic can be used in any case where the body is in need of detoxification or cleansing. Throughout the world, garlic is known to ease a plethora of ailments, from a weak metabolism, bad circulation and joint pain, to intestinal worms, respiratory infections and fevers. It has been shown in recent studies to have pronounced anti-cancer and anti-tumor effects. It is used to regulate both high and low blood pressure, as well as help to lower cholesterol.

Used externally, it is a fine antifungal and antiseptic treatment. This ancient food and medicine is valuable to relieve intestinal parasites, and possesses sufficient antibiotic strength to help treat severe infections.

There have been concerns lately among pet owners and veterinarian about the toxicity of garlic to pets. Onions and garlic both contain the chemical thiosulphate, which when consumed in large amounts can cause red blood cells to burst, causing a deadly type of anemia if left untreated. The general consensus among experts is that while onion is very dangerous (whether in small or large doses) to cats, dogs and even large livestock, garlic is safe in normal dosages. Garlic only presents a problem when given in very large doses.

Note: If you notice your pet is breathless or developing pale gums and tongue, than remove the garlic from its diet, as those are both signs of haemolytic anemia. The animal should restore its iron stores quickly and return to normal. Because cats have especially sensitive systems, garlic should only be given to them when needed, not on a regular basis, and certainly never in large doses.

Ginger

Zingiber officinale

Parts Used: rhizome

Properties: anodyne, antiseptic, carminative, digestive, hepatic, stimulant, tonic.

Ginger was first cultivated in China, and spread through Asia to Africa, and eventually the Caribbean. It is used extensively to calm digestive disorders, stimulating digestive enzymes and soothing the nervous system in that area of the body. The most common use for ginger with pets is to prevent nausea, with many owners claiming that ginger given before car-rides to dogs prevents motion sickness. Many dogs enjoy the taste of crystallized ginger, ginger soaked in a sugar solution and then dried.

Ginger is also used by many herbalists as a blood cleanser, and a general restorative tonic for the entire body, especially the circulatory system. It is believed to help heart disease and lower cholesterol. It is an anti-coagulant, and should not be used with animals that have low clotting factors or before surgeries.

Scientific studies have shown that ginger is a potent anti-inflammatory rivaling most conventional over-the-counter remedies. Ginger also seems to benefit diabetes in rodent studies. Recently, it has gained attention as a potential cancer adjunct.

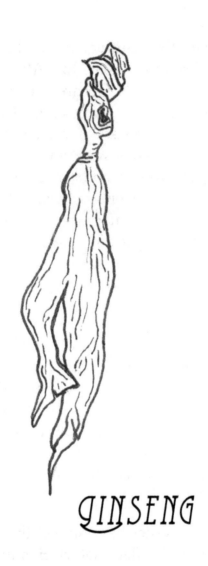

GINSENG

Ginseng, Korean

Panax ginseng

Parts Used: root

Properties: alterative, anti-carcinogenic, anti-oxidant, demulcent, immuno-stimulant, stimulant, tonic

Known in China as the "Root of Life", Korean Panax Ginseng is unparalleled by other ginsengs in its ability to strengthen and energize the entire body. Ginseng is useful for bolstering the immune system, in the treatment of Lyme Disease, arthritis, and any otherwise weakened condition. Lethargic, malnourished, depressed and abused horses are all generally good candidates for remedies containing ginseng. As they age, horses will have a better chance at longevity with a bit of ginseng added to their regular diet.

Ginseng is used to help prevent cancer cell replication, and has wonderful anti-oxidant properties. . Written around 100 B.C. in China, *The Herbal Classic of the Divine Ploughman* mentions ginseng's ability to fortify the body and fight cancer.

Modern western science is finally catching up with Eastern medicine, and studies have found that ginseng derivatives do in fact improve the survival and recovery rates chances of animals stricken with cancer. Furthermore, studies have shown that red ginseng is more potent than white ginseng on all fronts.

This herb is extensively cultivated, along with the other species, and is one of the most popular in Chinese, Japanese, Korean, and Russian traditional medicines. American ginseng, *Panax quinquefolium,* is good tonifying the lungs. Siberian Ginseng, or *Eleutherococcus senticosus,* is not a true ginseng as all, and is now generally called Eleuthero. Also an adaptogen, Eleuthero works very well to strengthen the immune system and stimulate mental faculties.

Goldenrod

Solidago canadensis

Parts Used: leaves

Properties: antioxidant, astringent, carminative, diaphoretic, diuretic, stimulant

Many animals, especially horses, love the anise-like flavor of goldenrod, and it can be used to enhance an herbal mixture's appeal when appropriate. Perhaps in part because of its sweet nature, goldenrod works well to strengthen the stomach and help prevent colic and flatulence. Often wrongly accused of causing seasonal pollen allergies, goldenrod can in fact help alleviate them, significantly reducing runny noses, asthma and other respiratory issues. Goldenrod's saponins act specifically against yeast and fungal infections, even common problems like cystitis, and can help break up and relieve bladder and kidney stones. Its diuretic action cleanses the kidneys and urinary tract.

In traditional European medicine, goldenrod is recognized as "a sovereign wound-herb, inferior to none, both for inward and outward use," according to Culpepper. It can be used externally to wash and heal wounds and burns.

Goldenseal

Hydrastis candensis

Parts Used: rhizome

Properties: antibiotic, antiseptic

Prized for its vivid yellow hues, goldenseal was used by Native Americans to treat wounds and make dyes. European settlers quickly learned from the local populace and further experimented with the root, finding it effective in the treatment of many kinds of infections, both internal and external.

Containing both hydrastine and berberine alkaloids, goldenseal can lower blood pressure and act as a mild sedative. Berberine has been shown in studies to kill tumors and parasites. Similar to prescription antibiotics, goldenseal can kill both good and bad bacteria in the digestive tract, and should generally be used in conjunction with a good probiotic to ensure digestive harmony.

Hawthorn

Crataegus oxyacantha, C. laevigata & C. monogyna

Parts Used: berries, flowers, leaves

Properties: astringent, antidiarrhetic, antioxidant, antispasmodic, cardiotonic, digestant, sedative, tonic.

Hawthorn is a well-reputed remedy for all things relating to the heart and circulatory system, and has been used by Native Americans in this capacity, as well as to treat arthritis and muscle soreness. Scientific animal studies have shown that it is an antioxidant with the ability to fight free radicals in the body.

Hawthorn strengthens and helps heal damaged collagen in the tendons and ligaments, offsetting the damaging effects of arthritic inflammation. In modern herbalism, hawthorn is used to treat heart murmurs and irregularities, both low and high blood pressure, pulmonary inflammation and heart disease, strengthening the heartbeat, and many studies have confirmed its efficacy.

The Chinese have long used hawthorn berries to alleviate poor digestion derived from circulatory troubles: used regularly in small doses, Hawthorn will gently improve circulation throughout the entire body. Animal studies have shown that it also prevents plaque buildup in blood vessels, and that tinctures from the berries lower cholesterol levels.

Horsetail

Equisetum arvense

Parts Used: leaves, stems

Properties: antibiotic, astringent, diuretic, styptic

Also known as bottlebrush and shavegrass, horsetail is a member of the ancient family of immense flora that dominated the earth some 400 million years ago. Lucky for us, it is fairly common, and has chosen to stick around, sharing its invaluable medicinal qualities. In South America, the tallest of these 30 unique species *E. giganteum*, can grow to a height of 30 feet.

Horsetail contains large amounts of silica and is extremely beneficial to horses in cases of skin allergies and suppressed urination. It has been shown by scientists to help bone and collagen formation, as well as calcium allocation in the body. Because of this, horsetail can also be used in any treatment that is designed to develop healthy hooves, bones or joints.

A decoction of horsetail added to a brace or salve can benefit slow-healing sprains and fractures, and relieve some skin conditions, especially eczema. Native Americans used horsetail rush to treat their horses' chronic swelling of the legs, rheumatic and arthritic problems, and to help speed repair of damaged connective tissue, improving natural elasticity.

Horsetail contains aconitic acid and can be used in both teas and washes to stop internal or external bleeding, thus a fine styptic, as well as to help rebuild damaged kidneys and livers.

Note: Do not use horsetail for more than six weeks without the proper herbal complements, as this herb may cause irritation in the digestive tract. Horsetail should not be used during pregnancy. A relative of horsetail, *Equisetum palustre*, has been shown to be toxic to horses, and should never be used in herbal applications.

Kelp

Laminaria digitata, Laminaria. saccharina

Parts Used: all

Properties: demulcent, emollient, diuretic, nutritive, tonic.

Kelp, or sea algae have long been used by Native Americans as foods and soothing medicines, especially to treat rheumatism, sore ligaments and muscles. Kelpswas used as winter feed for Native Americans' horses and cattle, and to treat a host of problems for both human and beast.

Kelp is a fabulous source of iodine, alkali, calcium silicon and contains many trace elements. Use as a general digestive aid and nutritional supplement, and to improve blood and hoof quality. In the winter, a bit of kelp in a horse's feed may encourage hydration and act as a deterrent against colic. Contemporary scientific evidence shows that sea algaes contain polysaccharides and minerals (especially iodine) that are immune stimulants.

Researchers have found that kelp is useful in regulating the thyroid, as well as deterring flea and tick infestations.

Licorice

Glycyrrhiza glabra

Parts Used: root

Properties: anti-inflammatory, demulcent, digestive, expectorant, immuno-stimulant, tonic.

Licorice, or sweet root, has been used throughout the ages for a wide variety of treatments. These days, its compounds have been analyzed by modern science and been found to be similarly beneficial. Licorice has been shown in animal studies to help ulcers, reflux and digestive issues, as well as heart disease, weight loss, and immune deficiencies.

Deglycyrrhizinated licorice, or DGL, is sold in many health food stores and is preferred by some herbalists over unaltered licorice for long term use: DGL does not deplete potassium stores, whereas licorice used long-term will, necessitating potassium supplementation when taken for more than a week. However, when using licorice to improve adrenal function, the herb is recommended over DGL, as it is the the glycyrrhizin which stimulates them.

Note: Licorice may have slight estrogenic effects, and is believed by some to be abortive: it is not recommended for use with pregnant or nursing animals.

Marshmallow

Althea Officinalis

Parts Used: root, leaves; whole plant

Properties: alterative, anti-inflammatory, demulcent, diuretic, emollient, expectorant, galactogogue, laxative, tonic, vulnerary.

The Greek word *Althea* means, "to heal" and the herb has provided countless medicines since ancient times. The emperor Charlemagne (742-814 A.D.) appreciated marshmallow and ordered it to be cultivated. Native to Europe and Asia, marshmallow was introduced to the Ancient Egyptians from Syria, where it was used to treat gastric disorders. Easing digestion, marshmallow has the ability to soothe and rehabilitate the kidney, colon and urinary tract with its lubricating properties. Similarly, it may be used to alleviate colic and diarrhea.

Marshmallow also has anti-inflammatory properties, and is extremely useful in the treatment of muscle and joint problems. It ameliorates lung irritations, coughs and dry, itchy nasal passages. Externally, a strong marshmallow infusion soothes and heals burns and abcesses.

A very safe, gentle herb, it is recommended for stimulating the production of milk in nursing animals. Do not feed to animals during pregnancy, as marshmallow can induce labor.

Meadowsweet

Filipendula (Spiroea) ulmaria

Parts Used: leaves & flowering tops

Properties: anodyne, febrifuge, anti-inflammatory, antirheumatic, antiseptic, diurectic

Known as "meadwort" during the Middle Ages, then Queen of the Meadow, this tall graceful herb was sacred to the Druids, and a choice "strewing herb" inside residences. Meadowsweet was esteemed by herbalists throughout the ages for its pain-relieving qualities and abilities to reduce fevers and remedy flu symptoms. Its high tannin content and astringent qualities make isteffective in treating diarrhea and some urinary tract infections. Many herbalists recommend it to relieve heartburn and gastritis. Its major benefit may be to relieve acidity.

Meadowsweet contains salicylic acid, first identified and obtained in 1835, and as such is useful in the same cases one would employ aspirin: for fevers, aches and pains. Horses respond well to its gentle properties, and it combines well with white willow and chamomile as a remedy to chronic arthritis. Dogs can be given low doses of meadowsweet every other day, once you have ensured that animal has been off other medications for several days as combination with drugs such as acetomenophine may prove fatal.

Note: Salicylic acid stays in feline systems for 48-72 hours, and can build up to toxic levels quickly. It is better to err on the side of caution and refrain from admistering meadowsweet to cats.

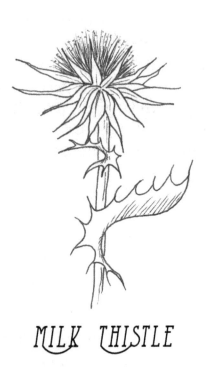

MILK THISTLE

Milk Thistle

Silybum marianum

Parts Used: seeds

Tall spiny biennial in the Daisy Family, **Compositae**

Properties: antidepressant, demulcent, galactagogue, hepatoprotective, tonic.

Milk thistle seeds, another Eurasian herb, contain *hesperidin* and *silymarin,* cell-strengthening antioxidants, and are the most powerful herb one can use to cleanse and treat liver. Milk thistle has been proven in clinical studies to significantly regenerate liver tissue. A potent preventative and corrective treatment for liver damage of any kind, milk thistle is, nonetheless, a safe herb for extended use. Just a couple of seeds a day will help protect the liver from toxins and help counteract the liver damage a horse may experience when on the stronger anti-inflammatory medications.

Milk thistle seeds are an excellent spring tonic and should be given for a month to 6 weeks, as the body absorbs their essence slowly. Grind the seeds well before adding them to the feed. This is especially good for horses and ponies that might be suffering from liver damage due to prolonged use of drugs, or from worming difficulties. Milk thistle can also improve appetite and help prevent colic, and was used for centuries in Europe by wet-nurses to improve their milk production.

Mullein

Verbascum thapsus

Parts Used: leaves & flowers

Properties: anodyne, astringent, antibacterial, antispasmodic, antiviral, demulcent, diuretic, emollient, expectorant, fungicide, pectoral, sedative, vulnerary.

Mullein is found throughout the United States, and its leaves were used by Native Americans to alleviate a variety of lung ailments, from whooping cough and bronchitis, to pneumonia, asthma, and influenza; leaves were applied externally as wound dressings. Mullein has a very mild sedative effect; this combined with its ability to expel mucus and remedy coughs makes it an invaluable treatment for seasonal allergies and chronic coughs. For a well-rounded respiratory treatment for head and chest colds, combine mullein with stinging nettle.

Mullein can also be used to treat pain associated with urination, and to help heal internal bleeding of the colon or diarrhea. Along with vitamin D and many B vitamins, Coumarin and Hesperidin are both found in Mullein, helping to strengthen veins and lending it a strong antioxidant effect.

Mullein is also reputed to expel tapeworms, though the authors have not tried this usage. Large concentrations of natural mucilage in this herb makes it a soothing expectorant. The yellow flowers in olive oil are a noted pain-relief remedy for earache. Externally, a warm poultice or salve made from mullein steeped in apple-cider vinegar will help bruises, pains and aches fade away.

Note: Mullein Seeds contain rotenone and are toxic to fish and insects.

Nettle, Stinging

Urtica dioica

Parts Used: leaves, roots, seeds

Properties: anti-inflammatory, astringent, diuretic, expectorant, galactagogue, hemostatic, nutritive, pectoral, tonic.

Nettle is one of the highest vegetable sources of iron and will restore the shine to an animal's coat. Nettles are a wonderful full-body tonic. Nettle Seed in particular is gaining popularity throughout the western world as a kidney tonic after several promising clinical trials. It has been shown to increase kidney function and treat renal failure with great success by bringing down harmful creatinine levels. As a diuretic and tonic, it cleanses and calm the kidneys and urinary system while raising an animal's overall Qi, or energy. During my own dog's second stab at acute renal failure in four years, a tiny pinch of seeds on her tongue every two hours along with IV fluids catalyzed a full and unexpected recovery.

Like mullein, another Eurasian herb in origin, nettle leaf and root are quite useful in most respiratory ailments, expelling mucus and easing congestion in both the lungs and sinuses. Nettle is an effective antihistamine, its own gentle histamines attaching to the body's receptor sites and preventing stronger allergic reactions. Stinging nettle leaf may also be a new therapeutic option for prolonging remission in inflammatory bowel disease, according to current research.

Rich in iron and potassium, stinging nettle is well-known throughout Europe for its ability to purify and tone blood and the circulatory system. Furthermore, its energizing and anti-inflammatory properties also make stinging nettle a valuable ingredient in any joint or arthritis therapy, and it has long been used both internally as a tea and externally as a poultice by Native Americans in this capacity.

To improve the quality of your pet's hair and to soothe sore muscles, make a strong infusion of stinging nettles and use it as a bracing rinse at the end of bathing.

Stinging nettles, along with red raspberry, are an ideal supplement to a pregnant animal's diet, providing many of the vital nutrients she needs. In particular, nettles are very high in vitamin K, which is very important for young mammals' proper growth and development.

Note: Occasionally animals can break

out in a slight "nettle rash" of raised bumps just under the skin; this normally disappears within 8 to 24-hours without problem. If your animal shows discomfort, discontinue use of nettles.

Oregon Grape

Mahonia aquifolium

Parts Used: Root

Properties: antibacterial, anti-fungal, antimicrobial, antiviral.

Oregon Grape root contains high levels of berberine, and for that reason is often used interchangeably with Goldenseal. Also for this reason, some botanists place it in the same class as Barberry, naming it *Berberis Aquifolium*. Recent studies have shown the Oregon Grape root decreases bacterial resistance to antibiotics in addition to its own efficacy as an anti-bacterial, and is used widely by herbalists to treat giardia, candida, diarrhea, and other viral or bacterial diseases. Both externally and internally, it can be very helpful in treating mange and other skin infections. Currently, it is receiving quite a bit of attention for its possible uses as an anti-cancer agent.

Peppermint

Mentha piperita

Parts Used: leaves

Properties: alterative, aromatic, calmative, carminative, diaphoretic, stomachic.

Peppermint was cultivated in Egyptian gardens in ancient times, and continues to be drunk as a tea in the Middle East for its digestive and cooling properties. Indeed, it has been used in the Middle East as a healing herb for over 3000 years, and was one of the favored herbs of physician Abu Mansur Mowafik, who wrote a treatise on pharmacology 1600 years before the birth of Christ. These same properties make it a natural remedy for colds, fevers, and flus. Grandmothers throughout the world know that a bit of peppermint in a cup of tea or a bowl of rice is guaranteed to bring some relief to a little one's upset tummy or fever, soothing cramps and nausea: and people aren't the only mammals who appreciate this tasty remedy. This is an herb that is well-loved by horses when dried, and can be added daily to a horse's feed to support proper digestion and help prevent colic.

Plantain

Plantago major

Parts Used: leaves and seeds

Properties: alterative, anti-inflammatory, antiseptic, astringent, diuretic, emollient, expectorant, refrigerant, vulnerary.

Plantain is another herb brought by the early settlers to America in the 1600s because of its many uses. The eastern Indians called it "white man's foot" because it so quickly spread everywhere the settlers went, and most native tribal herbalists were quick to apply its many therapeutic benefits. Perhaps its most important use is that when crushed into a poultice it has the fantastic ability to heal all manner of skin injuries. It can draw out the poisons from insect and spider bites, and quickly relieves burns, cuts and wounds. As an antiseptic, its anti-microbial properties will keep a wound clean, in addition to cooling the skin and soothing the pain. Infuse olive oil with bruised plantain leaves for two weeks and make a salve out of it to speed healing on all your animal's wounds and hotspots.

Taken internally, plantain's diuretic properties make it useful in treating urinary and digestive tract infections, as well as colic. Its demulcent and anti-inflammatory properties go far in soothing internal mucus membranes, too. Traditionally, it has also been used to treat cancer, and new studies are confirming plantain's effectiveness against viruses.

Prickly Ash

Xanthoxylum americana

Parts Used: bark

Properties: anodyne, circulatory, digestive, nervine.

Prickly Ash bark is a wonderful circulatory stimulant, helping blood flow particularly to and from the extremities. This makes it very useful in cases of gout, navicular, or arthritis in the limbs, where it acts as a carrier to help ensure that the herbs you are using actually reach toes, feet and tails.

Prickly ash can also be used as a rinse to help ameliorate tooth pain (it has a numbing effect inside the mouth) and as a digestive herb.

Note: Not for use in pregnant animals.

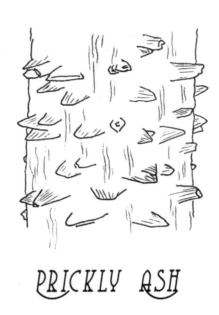

PRICKLY ASH

Raspberry

Rubus idaeus

Parts Used: leaves

Properties: alterative, antispasmodic, astringent, hemostatic, parturient, stimulant, tonic.

Raspberry is one of the few herbs that is not only safe for a pregnant animal to eat, but often recommended in small, regular doses by many herbalists as it can help prevent miscarriage and is reputed to ease birthing by strengthening the uterine muscles. Indeed, it is also beneficial during the menstrual cycle, easing cramps and calming the vaginal muscles.

As a hemostatic, is will prevent excessive bleeding in many situations, and can also be used to calm diarrhea. In Russian folk medicine, a decoction of the leaves is used as a cold and congestion remedy. Numerous Native American species of raspberries and their close relatives were used regionally by native people for foods and the therapeutic leaves and root bark served to treat everything from sore eyes and topical wounds, to easing childbirth and treating cancerous tumors.

Red Root

Ceanothus americanus

Parts Used: leaves

Properties: astringent, antispasmodic, expectorant, , lymphatic tonic.

Red root stimulates the lymph glands and helps clear extraneous fluid from the body. In this way, it is very beneficial to various cysts and most presentations of mastitis. It helps the blood move more effeciently, resolving issues with sluggish circulation and increasing blood charge.

Note: Red root should not be used on felines due to possible metabolic effects, or on seriously debilitated animals whose systems need to be strengthened, rather than stimulated.

ROSEHIP

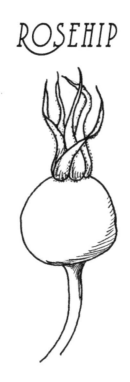

Rose hips

Rosa canina, R. rugosa

Parts Used: fruit

Properties: anti-cancer, anti-inflammatory, anti-oxidant, diuretic, laxative, nutritive, tonic.

Nearly all rose varieties produce rose hips, the round, hard tangy fruit after a rose flowers, but only a few varieties are used medicinally due to their superior flavor and medicinal properties. Dried rose hips are a great source caratenoids and vitamin C, containing more of the latter than citrus fruits by dry weight. They have shown significant results as anti-inflammatories combating joint pain and Osteoperosis in European trials, and contain phytochemicals known to actively fight cancer.

Saint John's Wort

Hypericum perforatum

Parts Used: leaves and flowers

Properties: anodyne, anti-inflammatory, anti-depressive, anti-microbial, anti-viral, astringent, expectorant, nervine.

St. John's Wort is known to many people for its well-documented uses as an anti-depressant, rivaling many patented drugs for its efficacy. It is lesser known, but no less effective, at boosting the nervous system and lessening nerve pain. Initial studies have confirmed this, and it is often used by herbalists both internally and externally to help with muscle soreness or localized nerve issues.

Science has also shown that St. John's Wort has significant anti-viral properties, making it a potent herb to keep in one's cabinet.

Note: St. John's Wort can cause temporary photo-sensitivity when consumed in large quantities, or when applied directly to the skin as a salve. Do not use in conjunction with other anti-depressants.

Saw Palmetto

Serenoa Repens

Parts Used: berries

Properties: anabolic, hormone regulation.

Saw Palmetto alters the effect of testoterone on the prostate gland, lessening the symptoms of benign prostate enlargement, and can help male animals combat frequent urges to urinate as well as painful urination. Some claims have been made that it may also increase sperm production, but this has not been proved in scientific studies.

Saw palmetto can be used to tone and strengthen male and female reproductive organs, as well as to help lean or debilitated animals build their strength and put on weight.

Note: Diarrhea occurs rarely with the use of saw palmetto. If this happens, cut back the dosage or discontinue use.

SCULLCAP

Scullcap

Scutellaria baicalensis

Parts Used:

Properties: anti-cancer, anti-inflammatory, anti-viral, sedative.

Scullcap is used throughout the world, but in different ways. In China and Japan, skullcap is generally used as an anti-viral agent, whose efficacy has been proven in clinical trials against the flu and various bacteria; it also inhibits tumor growth. In Japan, blood pressure has been lowered in animal studies with the use of skullcap, and throughout western herbalism it has been traditionally been used to sedate nervous conditions. It is also believed to be effective in treating epilepsy.

Note: Not for use in cats or in animals with compromised livers.

Slippery Elm

Ulmus fulva

Parts Used: inner bark

Properties: demulcent, expectorant, mucilaginous, nutritive.

Many people are familiar with slippery elm from its extensive use in throat lozenges. The inner bark of slippery elm is both delicious and nutritious, and indeed, slippery. In lozenges it will coat the throat and ease coughing. In teas, it's demulcent properties will reach the intestines and boost their beneficial mucous lining, reducing gastric distress and benefiting fistulas, IBS, diarrhea and more. Slippery elm powder can be made into porridge with a little warm water, and given to animals that are having a difficult time keeping food down or who have little appetite. The porridge, which is naturally sweet and has a mild taste reminiscent of maple syrup, is considered a wholesome, nutrient-rich food and was used extensively by Native Americans during winter months.

Slippery Elm is a soothing tonic for the entire body, and is very good taking orally by any animals recovering from internal surgeries, or used as a softening poultice on external scar tissue or dry, scaly skin. It has no known side effects, and can be taken for months when needed.

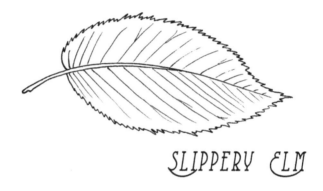

SLIPPERY ELM

Star Anise (Chinese)

Illicium verum

Parts used: seed

Properties: carminitive, stimulant, diuretic

Chinese Star Anise has long been used in Asia for colic and rheumatism. In more recent years it has gained popularity among herbalists as a potent anti-viral. Tamiflu is made from an extract of Star Anise, and many herbalists believe that a strong liquid extract of the seed will aid in zoonotic viruses such as SARS and Avian Influenza.

Note: Extreme care must be taken not to use Japanese Star Anise (Illicuim anisatum) which can cause severe neurological distress. Use on cats or on infants of any species is, for this reason, discouraged.

Thyme

Thymus vulgaris & species

Parts Used: leaves, stems, & blossoms

Properties: anodyne, antiseptic, antispasmodic, carminative, emmenagogue, expectorant, stimulant, respiratory tonic.

Thyme is extremely beneficial used in

all manner of headaches, emotional disorders, and sinus troubles. In the treatment of horses, it is a particularly valuable anti-inflammatory and mild pain-reliever for muscle and joint pains, and a general remedy for rheumatism. As it aids digestion and eases a variety of aches and pains, thyme can benefit almost any chronic discomfort.

Many species of thyme, each with different volatile oil contents, tannins, and flavonoids are used therapeutically to tonify internal organs and support the immune system. Thyme is a fine antiseptic tonic to treat respiratory problems, uterine buildup after birthing, and externally to treat spider and insect bites, thrush and other common fungal infections. Infusions of thyme are excellent to bathe horses.

Thyme was used throughout Europe in households as a favorite strewing herb, along with rosemary, sage and lavender. Scattered on the floor and walked upon, thyme's antiseptic properties discouraged disease while permeating the house with its gentle, pine-like fragrance; this is further enhanced by its insecticidal properties. Try sprinkling a bit among your animals bedding to bring in a bit of the outdoors.

Note: Being an emmenagogue, thyme is not recommended for use with pregnant animals.

Turmeric

Curcuma longa

Parts Used: rhizomes

Properties: anti-bacterial, anti-inflammatory, anti-tumor, antiseptic, digestive, stimulant.

Turmeric rhizome is familiar to many as the bright yellow powder used in Indian curries. In Ayurvedic medicine, it has long been used as an antiseptic and digestive remedy. More recently in the west its active component, curcumin has been identified with anti-cancer properties and as a potent anti-inflammatory. It stimulates the flow of bile and can be used to help gall-bladder and liver disorders.

It is also a good anti-bacterial agent, and can be used externally on wounds to speed healing (be careful, it stains!) and internally to fight infection. Studies in animals have also shown that it prevents LDL cholesterol build-up in arteries.

Uva Ursi

Arctostaphylos uva-ursi

Parts Used: leaves

Properties: anti-microbial, astringent, diuretic, tonic.

Known as bearberry among folk herbalists, Uva Ursi contains allantoin which soothes tissues and helps repair them. Containing hydroquinone and its derivatives, it is also one of the most beneficial herbs to use in bladder or kidney infections and disorders, clearing infections and relaxing the muscles so that they may heal. It helps remedy kidney stones and can relieve menstrual bloating and pain.

In addition to its traditional uses, Uva Ursi has recently been studied and found highly effective against E. Coli and other "bad" bacteria and fungi such as Candida Albicans and Enterrococcus faecalis.

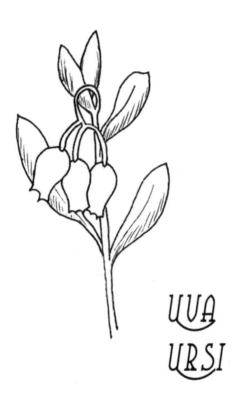

UVA URSI

Wheatgrass/Barleygrass

Triticum aestivum & Hordeum vulgare

Parts Used: young shoots and sprouts

Properties: anti-inflammatory, anti-oxidant, nutritive, tonic.

Wheat and barley grasses contain many vitamins and nutrients including B vitamins, vitamin C, vitamin E, calcium, potassium, iron and magnesium, and are considered by many to be a potent whole food. Animals love them, and even predator animals will eat grasses to stimulate digestion and gain enzymes for their stomachs. Both grasses carry proteins and compounds which are anti-inflammatory and act as a full body tonics. They also contain anti-oxidant cancer fighting enzymes that distinctly boost animal health.

Fresh is best with these grasses – grow them in a small tray for animals, and feed the cuttings or the juices. Or, buy the grasses in powder or tablet form, for ease of use.

White Willow

Salix Alba

Parts Used: bark & leaves

Properties: anodyne, anti-inflammatory, astringent, febrifuge, tonic.

Willow bark contains the glucoside *salicin*, that becomes *salicylic acid*, and is one of the original sources of aspirin, *acetylsalicylic acid*. In its herbal form, willow is a gentler, but often more effective therapy. As with aspirin, willow bark will reduce fevers, joint and muscle inflammation, and benefit the heart.

In European tradition, willow bark was used to treat gas and colic, as well as suppressed urine. Externally, willow may be added to braces or washes to hydrate and clean wounds, sores and burns. Native Americans used willow twigs as chew sticks and dentifrices to relieve toothache, and treat mouth and gum problems. This was also a fine source of vitamin C and other trace minerals. Native herbalists pounded willow bark into soothing poultices as wound dressings and to relieve joint pains for people, dogs, and horses alike. Native children knew the willows as the "headache trees" and the "toothbrush trees" favoring wet regions.

Note: Because it contains aspirin compounds, do not feed to felines.

Wild Indigo

Baptisia tinctoria

Parts Used: roots and leaves

Properties: antibacterial, anti-viral, immuno-stimulant, lymphatic.

Both modern research and historical usage have proven that Wild Indigo stimulates the immune system, and is a potent herb for use against all bacterial or viral infections. Use in small quantities, for short amounts of time, as larger quantities may induce vomiting and long-term safety has not been established. Wild indigo can also be used to restore health to the lymphatic system, and decrease glandular swelling.

Yarrow

Achillea millefollium

Parts Used: flowers, leaves

Properties: alterative, anti-bacterial, anti-spasmodic, astringent, carminative, diaphoretic, diuretic, hemostatic, tonic.

Yarrow is a great all-around herb, with cleansing and healing properties for the entire body, and is useful both internally and externally. Native Americans used yarrow to relieve chronic fatigue and weakness, as a wound dressing, and to stimulate circulation.

Yarrow was among the first herbs brought to America by our early ancestors, who had no way of knowing it already existed here. Internally, yarrow will cleanse the blood and strengthen many body organs, including the lungs. It helps purge toxins from the blood and kidneys, as well as bacteria and viruses from the body, making it extremely useful in the treatment of any cold or flu, and most childhood illnesses. It stops excessive bleeding, inside and out: use it to lessen excessive menstruation, heal internal injuries, and relieve bruises.

Externally, yarrow's ability to speed the clotting process makes it an ideal herb to heal all sorts of cuts and wounds. Simply make a tea or poultice of the dried herb or use fresh, slightly crushed, leaves and place directly on the wound to stem bleeding.

CHAPTER FOUR

Homeopathy & Flower Essences

"Our task must be to free ourselves...by widening our circle of compassion to embrace all living creatures and the whole of nature and its beauty."

~ Albert Einstein

What is Homeopathy?

Homeopathy is based on the idea that like cures like. The homeopathic practitioner uses a minute dose of something to cure the same: if you have poison ivy, you take rhus toxicodendron, poison ivy. What, you say? This sounds crazy, right. The idea is that you are an energetic being, and you are reacting to the poison ivy because energetically there is something in you that does not agree with the energy of the ivy. When you take it in miniscule doses, with purposeful intention, you are energetically signaling your body to get used to it. So if you are nauseous, your remedy is something that in conventional, herbalist dosages would make you vomit. But here's the trick: the dosage you are taking has been diluted so many times that there is *not one, single molecule* of the original organic matter present.

Homeopathic begin their life as full-strength "mother" tinctures, the same as you would make to treat someone herbally. To make it a homeopathic tincture, you place one drop of mother tincture in 100 drops of solution, shake the bottle and bang it on a table. This is step one. Homeopathic remedies come in many dosages, the most common being 6c, 30c, 200c and 1m, ranging from low to high doses respectively. The numbers indicate how many times the remedy has been diluted. So a 6c has been repeated step one **six times**. A 1m has been diluted **1000 times**. The more diluted the remedy, the stronger it is because each time the manufacturer intended to make it so, and agitated the molecules in the process activating the solution.

While it all sounds a little strange t o most Americans, homeopathy has a large and varied following, particularly in Europe where every pharmacy has a large homeopathic section, and most doctors are well versed in homeopathic remedies. Many doctors in the United States are beginning to prescribe Arnica homeopathic preparations before surgeries to reduce pain and recovery time.

I have found personal evidence of the efficacy of homeopathic remedies through animals and children. There is no question in my mind that they can and do work. Animals do not experience placebo effects when I place remedies in their drinking water, nor do young children and babies. They have no idea I've added anything "special" to their water. And so when they respond, I know it's real.

Basic Homeopathic Remedies for Animals

Most of the following remedies are available at local health food stores, as well as through mail order online. Some of the best companies are Boiron, NatraBio, Walsh, and Metagenics. Remedies are usually found in small pill forms or liquid dropper bottles. The pills are usually lactose or sucrose based, and very safe for all animals. Most animals will happily take these sweet, tiny pills orally. The tinctures generally contain alcohol, which animals will not like as much, but which can easily be added to drinking water or food.

Allium Cepa is used by people and animals alike for watery coughs, runny noses and eyes, and hay fever.

Arnica Montana can be taken either internally for generalized trauma or pain, or used topically as a gel or cream to treat local injuries. If used topically, make sure that the animal is not likely to lick it off, as few arnica creams are designed for ingestion.

Chamomilla is perfect for young animals who are teething or restless. Use it to help calm animals that are prone to stress or snapping. It is also indicated for inflammation and fever.

Ledum Palustre has been used in various clinical trials to treat Lyme disease in dogs with good results. Stephen Tobin, DVM, recommends "For treatment [of Lyme disease], I give one pellet of Ledum 1M three times a day for three days. I have been using Borrellia burgdorferi 60X nosode, a homeopathic preparation, as a preventative for Lyme disease in dogs. I give orally one dose daily for one week, then one dose a week for one month, then one dose every six months. One homeopathic MD runs titers on all his [human] Lyme disease patients, both before and after treatment with Ledum, and has found that there is a constant decline in titer after Ledum."

Hypericum is a must have for any animal 1st aid kit. It treats nerve injuries and shooting pains. Use for car accidents, puncture wounds, and spinal injuries. Hypericum is also indicated for nervous or depressed animals.

Nux Vomica helps control nausea, vomiting and diarrhea, making it useful for both illnesses and motion sickness.

There are hundreds of homeopathic remedies on the market. They come in both single formulations, like the ones listed above, and in mixed formulas containing multiple remedies for various illnesses or conditions. These mixed formulas are perfect if you don't know exactly what the cause of the condition is, because they will treat a multitude of symptoms and causes.

Modern Flower Essences

Flower essences are energetic infusions of flowers, made with water and preserved with alcohol, vinegar, or even vegetable glycerin. They work on very similar energy principles to homeopathy. Basically they are made from a much weaker mother solution and not diluted nearly as much as a homeopathic remedy. The first person to bring flower essences to market was the British surgeon Dr. Edward Bach, who came up with over thirty flower essences and created a combination formula called Rescue Remedy made from five of his essences to calm the mind and ease stress on the body and psyche. He found each of his remedies within walking distance of his country home, and used them to treat his own emotional disorders as well as the disorders of those around him.

These days there are many companies producing essences of many kinds: flowers, the environment, minerals, you name it. Flower essences are very simple to produce, and often the plants growing near you are the plants which will best heal you, as Dr. Bach discovered. Many herbalists believe that one need look no further than one's back yard for herbs: the same can hold true for flower essences.

Using Flower Essences

Flower essences work on similar principals to homeopathy, and as such cannot interfere with medication or exacerbate conditions. They can *only* improve a situation, never harm. Flower essences can be taken by the dropper-full under the tongue or in a glass of water. They may be placed next to the bed while you sleep or in your pocket during the day. Their beneficial harmonies are far-reaching, and do not need to be ingested to exert their happy influences. Try placing a few drops in the water bottle you carry throughout the day, or in your drink with dinner. Most importantly, use them with love and affection, for they will bloom under good attentions.

How Do I Choose a Flower?

Flower essences can be chosen based on what they do, and how they feel. Sometimes, they choose you. It is all right if you are not sure why you are drawn to a particular essence, or if the description of its uses does not align with the disorders you wish to treat. Each plant has more purposes than the small paragraph generally allotted to it on a website or in a brochure. Spend some time with different flower essence company catalogues, sorting the possibilities. Do not worry if the one you are drawn to does not list specific usages for pets. Flower essences can be used for all beings, great and small, to good effect.

Another way to choose a flower to work with is to meditate and quiet your mind, and ask for the flower to reveal itself. This is a wonderful way to connect with your own plants and flowers, find out what they are willing to help you with, and what they would like in return.

To begin, breathe in deeply, serenely. Breathe in, and breathe out. In and out. If you are not on the property whose guardians you wish to contact, take a few moments to imagine yourself there. Reach out with your mind's eye, and see your self in that space. Take some time to re-create the environment you wish to be in. Now, call out (silently in your head) to the flowers and fairies, the nature devas and the overlighting angels, your guides or your higher self, or who ever you wish to speak with. Perhaps you want the advice of the local fairy king, or the spirit of your climbing roses. Perhaps you wish to speak with your tomatoes and find out what effect their flowers have. Invite them in, whoever they are, and thank them for their presence and divine guidance. Tell them what it is you are seeking to know, or what you need help with. They will answer you, sometimes quickly, sometimes slowly. Be patient, and grateful for their loving, enduring guardianship of the land where you dwell.

Sometimes you may not connect with the plant itself, but the spirit of all peas, or all sunflowers. This is called a deva. Or you may connect with an overlighting landscape angel. Devas and angels watch over the land and the earth. They play with the wind and the trees, the skies and the waters. Devas are more intimately involved in the workings of the nature of the earth, it is they that the fairies and gnomes patterned themselves after when they decided to become less physical, and more non-physical, and to become more ONE with the energy play of the earth and the devas. Devas have been called nature spirits, sprites and sylphs for many years.

Overlighting angels are a bit more removed. They watch, and they help channel energy to the areas they watch. They speak with the devas and feel empathy for all living creatures in their area but they do not intervene on a physical level as much as the fairies or the devas. They will and do help the devas and the humans clear negative energy from areas when they are called in, and they do help connect humanity to Source. But they do not shift the winds or the rains or the sun or make the plants grow swifter or taller. That is the work and the play of the devas and the fairies. Every piece of earth has an overlighting angel. Some watch small areas of earth, and some watch very large pieces of earth. Most pieces of earth have several overlighting angels watching over them, at different levels, feeling different levels of connection and interpersonal connectedness. So, as your home or street has an overlighting angel, so does your city, and the general area of your state, and the area of your country, and also your entire country. Your entire planet has an overlighting angel called the Sun, and also the Moon.

Devas and angels can be called upon to help re-connect you to the earth or other elements of nature such as the sun, moon, plants or animals. They are particularly attuned to clearing spaces, large or small. Call on overlighting angels to clear geopathic stress, or energetic disturbances in mass consciousness. Devas are great for shutting down black streams of negative energy on your property, negative vortexes or portals to other planes and dimensions. Think about the size of space you want to clean, and then call in the appropriate nature spirit(s). Always ask them respectfully for their help, they do not appreciate being ordered around, but are eager to assist us in any way they can, so long as our motives and our intent are pure.

Be as clear as you can about what you would like them to do, and within minutes, days or weeks, depending on the job you set them to, you will see marked improvements. A simple and heartfelt "Thank You" is always appreciated when you are finished. Ask if there is anything you can do in return or addition to what they are doing: sometimes you may be asked to put a specific crystal somewhere, or plant a new flower. They may ask you to take a bath in saltwater, or you may hear nothing. All responses are ok. Even if you can not hear the fairies or the angels when they speak to you, trust that they are there, and they *do* hear you! Joyfully, lovingly, for their hearts are pure, they seek to help humanity heal itself and heal the planet around them.

Making Your Own Flower Essences

Flower essences are made by filling a clean glass jar or container with pure spring water. Float the flower gently on the water, or, if the flower is from a toxic plant such as foxglove, cover the container with its lid and then place the flower on top. Either way, the container should be covered and then placed in the sun for several hours.

If you wish, you can place clear quartz crystals around the container for further empowerment. When you are ready, remove the lid and the flower, and store the water in a dark glass container, mixed with vinegar (white or apple cider) in a 50/50 solution. Vodka or Brandy may also be used. If in doubt, ask your local devas, overlighting angels, or fairies for their advice. This solution is called the "mother essence". Any extra, unused essence water can be used to water you plants to great advantage.

When you wish to make dosage bottles for using the flower essence, choose glass, colored bottles (generally amber, blue or green) with droppers. Fill each bottle with ¼ vinegar and ¾ pure spring water, and add 12 drops of mother essence per ounce. If you are making a combination bottle which will hold multiple essences, add 3 drops per ounce of each mother essence. Working on an energetic level, flower essences remain dormant until they are needed, so that whichever ones are relevant at the time a combination formula is taken will be activated and work for the user.

Flower Essences for Animals

Allium is a flower of expansion and growth and alleviates fears. It frees animals from constrictions, and is good for expectant parents, during periods of change, and new situations.

Astilbe heals trauma and assists with the process of letting go. It is very good to clear away patterns of addiction, victimization, and abuse. Particularly good for rescue animals.

Black-eyed Susan reaches into the past to create a new lineage and heal familial rifts. It clears karma and heals anger and guilt. It uplifts the dark, and transmutes it to Light. Great for animals who may suffer from genetic behavioral problems, and pack in-fighting and anger issues.

Bleeding Heart is good for animals who have been abused, abandoned, or grieving the loss of a companion. It is also very beneficial for pregnant animals.

Bull Thistle allows one to see problems and issues that are hidden and locked away deep within themselves, so that one can release and transmute them positively. Physically, it boosts the immune system.

Clematis Flower essence fights tumors and growths in the body, and distortions of the mind. Ill thoughts, depression, and corruption all benefit from Clematis.

Clematis opens the higher chakras in short bursts, re-aligning them with their soul-purpose as they are cleansed. The mental and etheric bodies also benefit from Clematis, allowing miasms and karmic and genetic distortions to be re-programmed and wiped clean.

Evening Primrose balances the male and female aspects of the self, and also fosters easier relationships between the sexes. It encourages openness and honesty, truth and trust. Good for those who have a hard time entering relationships, as well as animals involved in breeding.

Flowering Raspberry draws the sweetness of life to oneself. It revitalizes the mind and clears "fuzzy" thinking. Benefits aging animals and people.

Foxglove is for healing any trauma in the past future or present. It heals wounds on all levels. It opens the heart for healing and shields from negativity. It lends strong, supple resilience to those who take it.

Gladiolus activates the kundalini and fires the soul, raising the vibration of the body simultaneously. It clears mass consciousness, facilitates transition and enables ascension. Helpful for auto-immune diseases and fatigue.

Hollyhock clears and connects all chakras in all the bodies: etheric, astral, physical, spiritual, mental. It allows one's life path to blossom and unfold as it was intended. Very healing to all physical issues, including chronic disease and allergies.

Honeysuckle works on the physical to heal cancers and immune disorders. It repairs RNA and DNA and helps transistion the body into a LIGHT-body, a crystalline form.

Hosta brings deep wisdom from the divine. It connects one to higher sources of knowledge and brings aged wisdom to animals who act a bit "goofy" or "spacey."

Joseph's Coat Climbing Rose aids in transitions of all kinds, and helps one allow miracles into one's life. It is a major energizer physically, facilitating the healing process.

Wild Lavender Bee-Balm relaxes the soul and allows one to let go of the stress of everyday life. It encourages "being in the moment," fostering patience and peacefulness. Great for overactive or nervous animals/people.

Miniature Red Rose helps one see the big picture. It brings a love of all things to the heart, and expands the heart chakra. It is pure love. Brings love to those in need. Great essence for nervous or aggressive toy breeds.

Mountain Laurel blocks geopathic stress and encourages resilience. It is the essence to use during epidemics and disasters to heal the heart and strengthen the psychic shield. It brings in the protection of the angels. Anytime one is in a new situation and needs a little boost of confidence, this a good essence to use. Wonderful for children or animals suffering from separation anxiety or feeling bullied others.

Mullein It clears away mental debris and silences inner chatter so that one can "hear" the big picture. Healing for ear problems.

Red Rose Climbing heals by blessing one with the Holy Spirit. It connects one to Source energy, reminding animals that they are all One, and part of the "pack."

Rose of Sharon connects you to Christ energy. The joy contained in this flower is ever blossoming, never fading. It lifts you up in times of sadness and reminds you of the Oneness of all things. Clears guilt and anger, restores purity of heart. Good for both the abused and the abuser. Top of Form

Sage helps animals transition into their advanced years gracefully, helping hair, bones and muscle retain youthful qualities. It also helps young animals assimilate into packs or herds, and calms overactive animals.

Squash Blossom frees animals. It pumps up their aura, larger larger largest. It gives them the strength to be themselves. Wonderfully healing for the shy and scared.

Strawberry Candy Daylily reminds one to delight in everyday, ordinary moments. It heals reproductive organs and traumas, and also re-creates familial bonds in a more positive way.

Tiger Lily shows that there is wisdom in folly, strength in laughter, truth in joy. It helps one let go of disapproval and feelings of inadequacy, and reminds us that we are all unique and necessary in the grand design, the Divine Tapestry of Life. Also good for digestive issues, and alpha animals that are too tough or dominant.

Weeping Wiegela allows genetic lineages to be cleared and healed as if they never existed, benefiting genetic and "incurable" diseases, also depression.

White Shasta Daisy bring out the wild, childlike joy in animals. It creates good bonds with children, for then they can see how they see. It restores innocence and purity. Helpful for childhood illnesses and traumas, as well as for aging.

Yellow Coreopsis is Joy and Laughter, and alleviates stress and worry. It also works with the digestive and urinary systems, and is very good for nerve or stress disorders.

CHAPTER FIVE

Essential Oils for Your Pet

"Just living is not enough... One must have sunshine, freedom, and a little flower." ~ Hans Christian Anderson

Essential oils are very concentrated extracts of the protective oils found in plant leaves, seeds and flowers. Sometimes, they are made from sap, or resins. Essential oils represent the first line of defense for many plants, and as such most are potent anti-bacterial and anti-fungal agents. Some of course, are stronger than others, but there are many overlapping uses for these oils.

As their name implies, most essential oil properties closely mirror the healing essence of their parent plants, in a concentrated form. It takes around four million jasmine flowers to create one pound of essential oil. Molecularly, essential oils are quite tiny, smaller than carrier oils, which allows them to absorb directly into the blood stream when applied to skin. Lavender, the herb recommended for sleep pillows and nighttime baby baths, yields an essential oil that is calming both for the mind and the body: lavender essential oil can speed healing and lessen pain. Horses are generally soothed by lavender, and we often put lavender on our wrists before riding.

Essential oils work on several levels. They can be diluted in a carrier oil and rubbed on the skin, or they can simply be spritzed in the air or on a cloth and inhaled. When essential oils are inhaled, they stimulate the olfactory receptor cells and transmit the cellular information of the oil properties to the limbic system, the emotional powerhouse of the brain, which is connected to the endocrine system of the body, as well as the respiratory and circulatory systems. From there, the information is transmitted to the entire body.

The modern practice of aromatherapy as we know it refers both to the inhalation and direct application of essential oils. A French chemist specializing in the creation of perfumes named René-Maurice Gattefossé was the first person to coin the term "aromatherapy." In a lab accident, he became intimately acquainted with the healing powers of lavender: burned in a fragrance lab explosion, he submerged his arm in lavender oil to dull the heat. He noticed that it also subdued his pain, and his arm seemed to heal faster than ever before. This spurred him on to further investigate the medicinal properties of essential oils, and in 1928 he published a book of his findings titled *"Aromatherapie."*

His work remained largely unknown, though it inspired a few adventurous doctors to experiment with his findings. In 1964, a French surgeon named Dr. Jean

Valnet published a book on essential oils by the same name as Gattefossé, covering his own experiments using oils to treat patients with emotional problems and physically-wounded soldiers during the second World War. The world was finally ready for *"Aromatherapie"* and the field has continued to grow and gain momentum as a valid medicinal treatment since its publication, with new research every year showing that essential oils have true medicinal value.

Carrier Oils

Many essential oils are too potent to be used full strength on the skin. Carrier oils allow essential oils to be applied directly to the skin. By diluting essential oils, which have extremely small molecules, with carrier oils, which have larger, fatty cells, essential oils may be used on the body. When applied directly to the body in a carrier oil, the smaller molecules of the essential oils are absorbed through the skin and reach the bloodstream within hours, or sometimes minutes depending on the oil being used. The carrier oil remains in the outer layers of the skin, acting as a harmless moisturizer.

It is very important to match your carrier oil to your specific needs. Carrier oils have different shelf lifes, thicknesses, odors, and even herbal properties. There are many oils on the market these days -- from the more common canola, soy, and sunflower to the lesser known walnut, grapeseed and more. In a pinch most oils will do, but there are six oils that are perhaps used the most in aromatherapy and massage work. These are: almond oil, apricot oil, avocado oil, grapeseed oil, jojoba oil and olive oil.

Almond and **apricot** are both very light oils, and absorb nicely when massaged into the skin. Their shelf life is the shortest of the six. A small amount of vitamin E added to your blend will extend the life of these oils without thickening them.

Avocado is quite rich and thick, and is fantastic for very dry skin, as is **olive** oil. Olive oil is an old favorite among herbalists due to its long shelf life and healing, nutritive properties. Olive oil can be stored for 12-18 months at room temperature.

Jojoba oil is one of the best oils for the skin. Solid at room temperature, it has an extremely long shelf life. Add it to your blends to increase shelf life and condition hair & skin. **Grapeseed** oil is a light oil with anti-inflammatory properties, making it the ideal carrier oil for liniments and wound salves.

Modern Extraction Methods

Choosing between different manufacturers of essential oils, and their different extraction methods, can be confusing. Make sure that all your essential oils are aromatherapy grade, and not just for fragrance use only. Even better, use food grade oils.

Essential oils today are generally extracted in one of four ways. Citrus seed extracts are generally made through cold-pressing. This means that the seeds are chopped and pressed, resulting in watery oil that has a shorter shelf-life than most essential oils, generally 6-8 months.

Many oils are made using solvent extraction, where the plant is mixed with a solvent. The solution distilled into a concentrated resin, which is combined with alcohol. The alcohol is allowed to evaporate, leaving behind the pure essential oil. When possible, avoid using oils extracted by this method. The solvents used often leave behind chemical traces of themselves, which can trigger reactions in people and animals, ranging from hives to allergies to depressed immune systems.

Most aromatherapists prefer to use oils extracted through steam distillation: no residues are left behind in this process, and they are considered more pure. Steam distillation extracts the essential oil in a still using pressurized steam. The steam carries the essential oils into a cooling pipe, where the vapors condense and the pure essential oils separate from the water.

The newest method of oil extraction is carbon dioxide extraction, which is quickly gaining popularity due to its simplicity and ability to produce pure, untainted essential oils. The plant is pressurized and turned into a liquid. When the chamber is depressurized, the carbon dioxide becomes a gas, leaving behind nothing but the pure essential oil. This method results in the most costly oils, though prices are slowly decreasing as more aromatherapists demand pure oils.

When choosing your oils, remember that animals are more sensitive to scents and chemicals than most humans. Choose the carrier oil that best suits its application. Take the time to find the best oils for your situation.

Essential Oils

Basil

Ocicum basilicum

Basil is uplifting and helps clear the mind. It is a very good herb to use in stressful situations and works wonders on viruses and nerve disorders. It can be used to benefit liver, kidney and urinary tract problems.

Benzoin

Styrax benzoin

A drop of bezoin in every ounce of salve or aromatherapy oil will prolong its shelf-life due to its potent antiseptic properties. Sticky and sweet, it is a natural wound dressing with a calm, relaxing effect on the psyche. Benzoin increases circulation, also making it useful in the treatment of aches and pains.

Calendula

Calendula Officinalis

Calendula one of the best herbs to take the time to prepare as an infused oil. It's gentle, calming and drawing nature will benefit any skin condition, from skin allergies and rashes, to dryness, bites and bruises.

Chamomile, German

Matricaria chamomilla

Similar to the herb, German chamomile oil has strong anti-inflammatory and anodyne properties, and will benefit muscle soreness, headaches and menstrual cramps. Apply a drop directly to swollen insect bites twice a day to reduce the pain.

Fennel

Foeniculum vulgare

Fennel oil is a mild painreliever and anti-inflammatory, which makes it very good for healing bruises, aches and pains. Fennel is a mild appetite suppressant that decreases bloating, making it a perfect addition to any weight loss program.

Geranium, Rose

Pelargonium graveolens

Throughout the Mediterranean you will find windowboxes filled with bright geraniums. Sure, they are pretty and easy to grow, but the real reason everyone plants them? Most European houses don't have window screens, and rose geraniums keep the mosquitos outside. Use the calming scent of geranium essential oil in sprays and on collars to keep biting insects away from animals in the summer

Rose Geranium is also unparalleled as a skin conditioner, with the possible exception of Myrrh, preferred by the ancient Greeks. Geranium oil can be used to treat wounds, burns, scars, bites, inflammations and infections.

Lavender

Lavandula angustifolia

As mentioned in the beginning of this chapter, lavender's anti-inflammatory and soothing properties gave birth to the science of aromatherapy. Used topically, lavender is not only a calming scent, but also a natural remedy for wounds, insect bites, rashes and burns; Add a couple drops every day to wound dressings to keep infection at bay.

In Europe, lavender was one of the four herbs used in the famous "Four Thieves Vinegar," so named for four men who tended the plague-afflicted for years without ever getting infected. They attributed their hardiness to the vinegar: every day before going out, the "four thieves" would drink a dram of the herb-infused vinegar, and wash their hands and faces in it upon returning home from the beds of the sick.

Lemon Eucalyptus

Eucalyptus citriodora

Eucalyptus is widely known for its lung- and sinus-clearing properties, as well as it cooling nature. Lemon eucalyptus works similarly, with a stronger citrus scent. It is a stronger anti-inflammatory and anti-bacterial than eucalyptus, which makes it a fabulous ingredient in any salve destined to treat minor wounds and bruises. A little goes a very long way with this one! Combined with rose geranium or opopanax, it will also help keep away biting insects.

Mugwort

Artemisia vulgaris

Mugwort-infused oil is wonderful for sore, tired muscles. The Natuve Americans used it like sage to purify spaces and keep minor wounds from becoming infected. In China, the oil is used to heal bruised areas.

Myrrh

Commiphora myrrha

Myrrh is arguably one of the most blessed resins: used to mummify the dead in Egypt and as a wound dressing in Ancient Greece by the Olympiads, and then given to Jesus as a babe in arms, myrrh has a grand history. Myrhh will ameliorate almost any skin problem, keep wounds closed and uninfected, and speed healing. Use it for saddle sores, minor wounds and bites, and dry, cracking skin. Added to tooth pastes or powders, it will benefit gums and teeth, alleviating soreness and acting as an antiseptic. Myrhh tinctures can also be taken internally to help fight sore throats and minor colds.

Opopanax

Illicium verum

The woody, musty scent of opopanax is one of the best, and indeed only, scents that really deter ticks. Add a several drops in with your daily fly spray bottle or place a few drops on your pet's collar to keep the hungry beasties away.

Rosemary

Rosemarinus officinalis

Any salve destined to treat inflammation and soreness simply *must* contain rosemary! Rosemary will produce a powerful liniment, heating and penetrating sore muscles and improving sluggish circulation. Rosemary can also be used to increase over-all energy, alertness and memory, and a sniff before training can help keep your animal alert and interested – although a good trainer knows that keeping it fun works best.

Sage

Salvia officinalis

Sage oil is both antioxidant and antiseptic, and will nip fungal infections in the bud. Sage can also be used to stimulate hair growth on saddle sores and mangy areas.

Note: Sage oil may reduce lactation in nursing mares.

Sandalwood

Santalum album

Sandalwood is one of the most popular scents in the world, and with good reason. In India, wet nurses are required to rub sandalwood paste on their breasts each day. Its gentle, calming scent treats soreness and nerve problems. It is also a good anti-inflammatory, making it a useful base note in both salves and liniments along with other oils.

Tea Tree

Melaleuca alternifolia

A member of the large and diverse eucalyptus family, tea tree is an extremely powerful antiseptic and anti-fungal oil. It can be used undiluted on most people and animals, but spot test first to make sure your animal is not sensitive to it. A few drops can be rubbed right on the skin onto insect bites to relieve itching and swelling, as well as applied to minor wounds to speed healing and deter infection.

Thyme

Thymus vulgaris

Similar to the dried herb, thyme oil is used as an anti-inflammatory pain reliever in liniments and salves to treat sore, tired muscles. Combined with rosemary, thyme oil creates a potent anti-inflammatory liniment.

Yarrow

Achillea millefolium

Yarrow-infused oil, particularly when combined with geranium or myrrh, is a wonderful balm for skin wounds and rashes, and can calm all manner of irritated skin. Plus, it smells heavenly.

Ylang-ylang

Cananga odorata

Known in the Far East for its ability to stimulate the growth of luxurious hair, ylang-ylang has been proven in western trials to control the production of scalp sebum, which is often a factor in slow hair growth, and even hair loss. Combine with sage for a great hair tonic, or with rosemary to condition and create shine.

CHAPTER SIX

Support from Mother Earth: *Crystal Healing*

"The land is sacred. These words are at the core of our being. The land is our mother, the rivers our blood."
~ Mary Brave Bird

Minerals have been used by healers for thousands of years. Crystals and rocks carry the soothing, grounding energy of the Earth within them. Each stone has a different crystalline structure which resonates at a difference frequency, and each frequency targets a different healing energy. Some crystals are used for healing, some for calming, some for joy and some for protection. Many great books exist about crystals: two of my favorites are "*The Crystal Bible*" by Judy Hall and "*Love is in the Earth*" by Melody. The first is a beautifully illustrated reference with all the most common stones, well-suited for beginners, and the second is a vast compendium of every stone ever named.

Supporting stones can be placed near your animal's sleeping area, in your animal's drinking water, worn around their neck or tied to their saddle. They can be placed near the animal when you are conducting hands-on healing work, or placed near your tinctures and remedies for empowerment. Used in the environment, crystals heal harmonic discord and can even ameliorate EMF waves. They are soothing and beneficial to all beings, on many levels.

Amethyst works with the brow chakra to help stimulate intuition, eyesight, and understanding. It can help boost animal communication, while fostering feelings of calm and acceptance. Physically, it can benefit eye and ear disorders, as well as head trauma.

Aquamarine, the stone of peace, can be used to help soothe wild or stressed animals. It also works on the throat chakra, increasing communication and diffusing anger.

Bloodstone is traditionally believed to be capable of miracle healings. Bloodstone is indeed a powerful healer, cleansing the blood, liver and reproductive systems, and is helpful in all dis-eases. It activates the root and heart chakras and draws energy from the earth directly through the legs and reproductive organs, dispersing energy equally throughout the entire body via the circulatory system and the meridians. It is a comforting, protective stone that brings calm and reassurance to the wearer, lowering the heart rate and blood pressure while soothing the soul.

Carnelian energizes the physical body and stimulates healthful activity while grounding. Excess energy from the upper chakras is transmuted by carnelian into physical strength and vitality. Negativity rolls off the back when one bears this stone, making the bearer impervious to ill will from others. This is a good stone for low-ranking, omega pack animals to wear on their collars. It helps heal wounds of the heart, blood and body.

Citrine brings the animal feelings of joy and contentment, and works on the third chakra to heal digestive, spleen and kidney troubles.

Danburite helps animals feel more comfortable in their bodies and has a particularly soothing, calming effect. It benefits all chakras and dis-eases.

Kyanite clears and aligns the chakras of

all those who come near it. When it is worn, it has a constant protective and grounding effect as it clears and aligns, clears and aligns, over and over again. The bearer of this stone is quite difficult to knock off-balance energetically. Because the chakras are aligned and open, one's higher self and energy body are able to enter the physical body, leading to higher ascension and attunements. Kyanite is easily found in many shades of blue and blue-green, as well as black: black Kyanite is more protective but less aligning than blue Kyanite.

Leopardskin Jasper allows one to get in touch with animals and the grounding forest/jungle aspect of the earth. It facilitates animal communication calls in the protection of the large cats to the wearer.

Malachite is the supreme stone for general physical healing. It also can help boost fertility. Because malachite is high in copper, it is not recommended to place this stone in drinking water: instead, use green agate, which has very similar properties.

Onyx can be found in many earthy colors, including brown, green, and black and has a warm, safe, feeling. The green can be mossy or brilliant, and is good for healing and connecting to nature. Brown onyx helps kundalini energy flow up and through the root chakra, strengthening the body and will, and remediating many reproductive issues. Black onyx is best for protection and courage.

Quartz, whether clear or white, can be used for practically any purpose. Quartz is energizing, clearing and strengthening, and can be used to empower any healing remedy.

Rose Quartz is the stone of unconditional, compassionate love. It is the best stone to use for traumatized animals. If your animal is going to be staying overnight at a vet's or a kennel, leave a piece of rose quartz with her to keep her company.

Selenite is a powerful clearing stone. A good-sized chuck placed in a room will clear any and all negative vibrations. Selenite is one of the few stones which is so good at clearing, it never needs to be cleansed itself. It simply cannot hold a lesser vibration, making it valuable in the removal of tumors, worms, entities and energy "vampires."

Smoky Quartz is a dependable grounding stone that also carries the clearing properties that open the crown chakra, allowing the dual energies of the earth and the higher realms to flow freely in and out of the body through both the crown and root chakras. Tibetan Smoky Quartz has the added benefit of carrying centuries of Buddhist prayer energy within it, helping to facilitate calm serenity in the face of adversity.

Tiger's Eye is a beautiful, striped stone of golds, browns, blacks and blues. Sometimes it takes the appearance of a hawk's eye, in which case it is believed to increase insight and understanding in the owner, and can be used to benefit healing work with birds. Golden Tiger's eye connects the holder to feline energy. All tiger's eye is very protective and helps protect travelers.

Topaz is a very high-vibration stone that comes in varied colors. The different colors are good for different things. Golden, or Imperial, topaz helps boost immunity and increase overall Qi energy within the body. Blue Topaz works with the throat to clear respiratory disorders and aid communication and empathy. Silver topaz clears the body of dis-ease and increases joy.

CHAPTER EIGHT

Ailments & Their Remedies

"The wish for healing has always been half of health."
~ Lucius Annaeus Seneca

Ailment	Herbs	Crystals	Oils
Aging	Astragalus, Bilberry, Cleavers, Red Clover, Dandelion, Ginseng, Hawthorn, Milk Thistle	Danburite, Kyanite	Geranium, Rosemary, Thyme

Allergies	Barberry, Calendula, Chamomile, Dandelion, Elecampane, Garlic, Goldenrod, Marshmallow Mullein, Nettles	Bloodstone, Kyanite	Yarrow
Anxiety	Borage, Chamomile, Red Clover, Mullein, Rosehips, Scullcap, St. John's, Yarrow, Willow	Aquamarine Citrine, Danburite, Quartz, Rose Quartz	Basil, Benzoin, Geranium, Lavender, Sandlewood
Appetite	Devil's Claw, Garlic, Ginger, Goldenrod, Kelp, Marshmallow Milk Thistle, Nettles, Peppermint	Citrine, Malachite	Fennel, Rosemary
Arthritis	Borage, Burdock, Chamomile, Cleavers, Comfrey leaves, Dandelion, Devil's Claw,	Bloodstone, Carnelian, Coral, Onyx, Smoky Quartz	Benzoin, Thyme, Chamomile Lavender, Mugwort, Rosemary, Sandlewood Thyme

	Hawthorn, Marshmallow Meadowsweet Nettles, Peppermint, Turmeric, Thyme, Willow		
Blood Cleansing	Burdock, Red Clover, Dandelion, Echinacea, Garlic, Ginger, Kelp, Milk Thistle, Nettles, Red Root, Yarrow	Bloodstone, Carnelian, Garnet	Tea Tree, Yarrow
Blood Pressure	Bilberry, Celery, Cleavers, Garlic, Ginger, Hawthorn, Willow	Bloodstone, Rose Quartz	Geranium, Lavender
Bones	Boneset, Kelp, Horsetail, Stinging Nettle, Comfrey Leaves, Horsetail	Coral	

Bruises	Borage, Cleavers, Devil's Claw, Meadowsweet Nettles, Thyme, Willow	Bloodstone, Carnelian, Magnetite Unakite	Calendula, Fennel, Lavender, Myrhh, Rosemary, Sandlewood Thyme
Cancer	Astragalus, Barberry, Burdock, Chaparral, Cleavers, Red Clover, Dandelion, Garlic, Ginseng, Milk Thistle, Plantain, Red Root, Willow, Yarrow	Bloodstone, Citrine, Selenite, Rose Quartz	Tea Tree
Circulation	Cleavers, Garlic, Hawthorn, Meadowsweet Mint, Nettles	Bloodstone, Carnelian	Benzoin, Rosemary
Colic	Apples, Bilberry, Chamomile, Cleavers, Goldenrod, Kelp, Marshmallow Milk Thistle, Peppermint, Slippery Elm, Willow	Citrine, Topaz	Basil, Fennel

Congest-ion	Red Clover, Elecampane, Garlic, Ginger, Marshmallow Mint, Mullein, Nettles, Thyme	Amethyst, Topaz	Lemon Eucalyptus
Constipa-tion	Apples, Boneset, Cleavers, Elder, Marshmallow Slippery Elm	Onyx	
Coughing	Borage, Burdock, Comfrey Leaves, Elderberry, Marshmallow Mullein, Slippery Elm	Aquamarine Citrine, Tiger's Eye	Eucalyptus
Dehydration	Burdock, Kelp, Marshmallow Nettles, Willow	Aquamarine	
Depress-ion	Borage, Chaste Tree, Ginseng, Peppermint, St. John's Wort	Citrine, Kyanite, Rose Quartz, Tiger's Eye	Basil, Geranium, L. Eucalyptus, Rosemary

Detoxification	Burdock, Dandelion, Garlic, Nettles, Yarrow	Bloodstone, Selenite	Basil
Diarrhea	Apples, Bilberry, Marshmallow	Onyx	
Digestion	Chamomile, Comfrey Leaves, Dandelion, Goldenrod, Peppermint, Licorice, Marshmallow Nettles,	Citrine	Basil, Fennel, Rosemary
Ears	Calendula, Garlic, Mullein	Amethyst, Selenite, Leopardskin Jasper	Lavender, Yarrow
Eyes	Bilberry, Marshmallow	Amethyst, Quartz	Peppermint
Fatigue	Astragalus, Elecampane, Ginseng, Licorice, Peppermint, Rosemary, Thyme, Yarrow	Carnelian, Citrine, Kyanite, Quartz	Lemon Eucalyptus, Rosemary,

Fear	Chamomile, Echinacea, Mullein, Yarrow	Carnelian, Onyx, Tiger's Eye	Basil, Benzoin, Chamomile Sandlewood
Fever	Boneset, Borage, Burdock, Chaparral, Garlic, Ginseng, Meadowsweet Peppermint, Willow, Yarrow	Amethyst, Aquamarine	Yarrow
Fleas	Calendula, Garlic, Mint, Thyme, Yarrow	Selenite	Chamomile, Geranium, Opopanax
Flies	Calendula, Garlic, Yarrow, Peppermint	Selenite	Geranium, Lemon Eucalyptus, Opopanax
Hair Care	Calendula, Horsetail, Kelp, Marshmallow Nettles, Plantain, Rosemary		Geranium, Lavender, Rosemary, Sandlewood Tea Tree, Ylang-Ylang

Hair Growth	Burdock, Horsetail, Kelp, Nettles, Peppermint	Leopardskin Jasper	Geranium, Rosemary, Sage, Ylang-Ylang
Heart	Elecampane, Hawthorn, Meadowsweet Willow	Carnelian, Rose Quartz	Benzoin, Rosemary, Sandlewood
Hooves and Nails	Cleavers, Calendula, Garlic, Horsetail, Kelp, Marshmallow Nettles, Plantain, Meadowsweet Prickly Ash, Willow, Yarrow	Onyx	Calendula, Geranium, Myrhh, Rosemary, Tea Tree
Hormones & Glands	Boneset, Borage, Chaste Tree, Red Clover, Red Root, Saw Palmetto		Fennel
Immune System	Boneset, Echinacea, Elecampane, Garlic, Ginseng, Willow, Thyme	Malachite, Kyanite	Lavender

Inflamm-ation	Boneset, Borage, Chamomile, Celery, Cleavers, Devil's Claw, Marshmallow Meadowsweet Nettles, Thyme, Willow	Smoky Quartz	Chamomile Lavender, Lemon Eucalyptus, Myrhh, Rosemary, Sandlewood, Thyme
Internal Bleeding	Horsetail, Raspberry Leaves, Yarrow	Bloodstone, Carnelian	Yarrow
Joints	Boneset, Borage, Burdock, Chamomile, Dandelion, Devil's Claw, Hawthorn, Horsetail, Marshmallow Meadowsweet Mint, Nettles, Thyme, Willow	Carnelian, Danburite	Chamomile Lavender, Rosemary, Sandlewood Thyme
Kidneys	Burdock, Dandelion, Goldenrod, Horsetail, Marshmallow Yarrow	Citrine, Topaz	Basil, Yarrow

Laminitis	Dandelion, Garlic, Kelp, Marshmallow Meadowsweet Nettles, Thyme, Turmeric, Willow	Onyx	Chamomile Lavender, Myrhh, Rosemary, Sandlewood
Liver	Bilberry, Dandelion, Horsetail, Milk Thistle	Bloodstone, Smoky Quartz	Basil, Yarrow
Lungs	Borage, Mullein, Nettles		
Lyme Disease	Garlic, Ginseng, Hawthorn, Kelp, Meadowsweet Nettles, Peppermint, Thyme, Willow	Leopardskin Jasper, Selenite	Basil, Lavender, Rosemary, Sandlewood Thyme
Menstru-ation	Chamomile, Chaste Tree, Kelp, Nettles, Thyme, Yarrow	Bloodstone, Onyx	Chamomile Yarrow
Minor Wounds & Bites	Bilberry, Calendula, Comfrey Leaves, Echinacea,	Malachite	Benzoin, Chamomile Lavender, Lemon Eucalyptus,

	Garlic, Goldenrod, Horsetail, Marshmallow Plantain, Raspberry Leaves, Thyme, Yarrow		Myrhh, Sandlewood Tea Tree, Yarrow
Navicular	Borage, Burdock, Chamomile, Comfrey Leaves, Devil's Claw, Hawthorn, Horsetail, Marshmallow Meadowsweet Mint, Nettles, Thyme, Willow	Bloodstone, Carnelian, Kyanite, Onyx	Chamomile Lavender, Rosemary, Sandlewood Thyme
Nervous	Chamomile, Corn Silk, Mullein, Scullcap, Yarrow, Willow	Aquamarine, Danburite, Kyanite, Onyx, Rose Quartz, Selenite, Smoky Quartz, Topaz	Basil, Benzoin, Geranium, Lavender, Sandlewood
Nursing	Chamomile, Chaste Tree, Dandelion, Fenugreek,	Rose Quartz, Danburite	Chamomile Fennel, Lavender

	Marshmallow Milk Thistle, Nettles, Raspberry Leaves, Rose Hips		
Nutrition	Red Clover, Kelp, Nettles, Raspberry Leaves, Rose Hips, Slippery Elm	Citrine	
Pain	Boneset, Chamomile, Devil's Claw, Meadowsweet Nettles, Thyme, Willow	Danburite	Benzoin, Chamomile Lavender, Mugwort, Rosemary, Sandlewood
Pregnancy	Nettles, Raspberry Leaves	Danburite, Pearl, Rose Quartz, Quartz	
Respirat-ory Tract	Borage, Chaparral, Comfrey Leaves, Elecampane, Marshmallow Mullein, Nettles, Thyme	Malachite	Lemon Eucalyptus

Skin Allergies & Rashes	Borage, Burdock, Calendula, Chaparral, Cleavers, Comfrey Leaves, Dandelion, Elecampane, Garlic, Horsetail, Marshmallow Nettles, Plantain, Yarrow	Danburite	Calendula, Geranium, Lavender, Sage
Snake Bite	Echinacea, Garlic, Plantain, Yarrow	Selenite	Lavender, Lemon Eucalyptus, Tea Tree
Ticks	Garlic, Thyme, Peppermint, Yarrow	Selenite	Basil, Chamomile Geranium, Opopanax
Tonic	Burdock, Celery, Chaparral, Red Clover, Comfrey Leaves, Dandelion, Ginseng, Nettles	Quartz	Basil, Rosemary, Yarrow

Urinary Tract	Celery, Cleavers, Dandelion, Goldenrod, Horsetail, Marshmallow Plantain, Willow, Uva Ursi, Yarrow	Aquamarine Carnelian, Onyx	Basil, Fennel
Worms	Black Walnut, Clove, Elecampane, Garlic, Mullein, Oregon Grape, Thyme, Wormwood	Selenite	Basil, Tea Tree, Thyme

CHAPTER NINE

Pet Communication & Care

"We are brothers and sisters with all living things on this earth. All the animals and fish and birds have red blood just like we do, they breathe the same air that we breathe, they drink the same water that we drink. That's why we call them our relatives. And that perspective needs to be brought out. It tells about us conveying some kind of knowledge or ability to at least somehow communicate with other species on this earth."~ Allen Pinkham, Nez Perce, 2002

There is a vast body of knowledge that shows that animals, just like humans, benefit from physical contact. Animals groom each other when they are upset or hurt, using body language and gestures that are intended to comfort. Felines, in particular, generate tissue-healing sound frequencies when they purr, so if you have an injured cat, do everything you can to encourage them to purr. In fact, research has shown that these sound waves travel quite well, so if your animal with injuries has a feline friend, let them be in the same room together as much as possible. (Von Muggenthaler)

Eastern and Western alternative health specialists believe that there is a universal energy that runs through all living matter, animating it. This is what gives plants the ability to communicate with each other and form defensive strategies against pests as one thinking, feeling organism, and why music effects their mood and their growth. In the East it is called Chi or Qi, and in Western mysticism it is called simply the soul. In modern physics, it is being measured and recognized that there is an energy pattern that flows through all beings. And so, we all respond to energy, recognizing in it a sympathetic resonance.

When we hug our children, we give them both physical, emotional and energetic comfort. And when we pet our animals, they connect directly to our energy, allowing our goodwill and love to flow directly into them, or conversely, from them to us. It is no secret that pet-owners have been found in studies to enjoy better health and longevity, as well as lower blood pressure and stress indicators.

Domesticated animals are, by and large, loving, forgiving creatures. They will withstand abuse and negligence in return for a modicum of attention. And given proper love and care, they will give us much, much, more. They yearn to share this with us – their love and appreciation. Would you like to communicate with your animal? Often all it requires is a little bit of peace and quiet, and intent.

Choose a quiet, peaceful time of day in a place where you will not be disturbed. Sit silently with your animal, stroking it if that is something it finds pleasing, and sending it feelings of love and appreciation for its companionship. Settle your mind. Allow it to go still, quiet. Empty. Ask your animal silently if there is anything it would like to share with you. Remain open and receptive to whatever images or "words" you receive.

Often, our animals do not communicate in a clear voice, as people do, but in shapes and colors, images. Give yourself intellectual leeway when you are interpreting your animals' messages, and remember that you are receiving thoughts from an animal's perspective, not a human's. Animals have full emotional capacity, but they are more connected to Source energy and the natural flow of life on earth than humans. So there is less distance from their emotions to their thoughts, and they are generally very, very straightforward.

They do not lie, or beat around the bush. They live life in direct contact with their own soul or higher self, while our ego is often stuck in the role of translator between body and soul. Be prepared to be surprised. Animals are the ultimate teachers for being in the moment, in the flow, tuned in and turned on.

Animals may not seem to need much, because they are always in the flow. God, Source, Universe – it is consistently responding to the animal's wishes and giving the animal what it wants. Animals do not fear death, and will almost always choose death over lingering in pain. They have come to Earth not to create, as humans have, but to experience and to support. They are fully experiencing the joy-full, expansion of the universe at all times.

This is not to say that our pets cannot benefit from our help and care. They have placed themselves in a position of dependency so that they may support us energetically and emotionally, and they rely upon us for food, love and shelter. When your animal is ill, it may benefit immensely from the alternative therapies mentioned in this book. But it will benefit most of all from hands-on-fur contact. Hold your animal. Send it thoughts of love and gratitude.

You do not need to be trained in the arts of **Reiki** or **Healing Touch** to heal your animal with your energy. All you need is the will.

The first animal I healed energetically was also the first animal I owned as an adult. Young and fit at three years old, Remus began moaning and yowling for the entire morning and afternoon. Something was very wrong. He was fevered, listless and I felt strongly that he was going to die – and my vet was on vacation. I planned to bring him to an emergency clinic first thing the following day. Distraught, I headed to my balcony that evening to drum and meditate, hoping to calm myself somewhat. Remus followed, and while I drummed a healing song entered my mind – the first I ever heard. Remus approached and curled up on my lap, and I sang, drummed, and cried, rocking him and channeling him my energy the whole time. After twenty minutes, I stopped and he sprang from my lap. No moaning. No yowling. Full of energy and vigor, it was like he was never sick.

I do not believe that you need to be specially trained or gifted psychically to heal your animal. We all have the ability to pass on the energy of well-being and joy to others. Reach a place of love, where you can connect to the highest good of the animal, and channel that intention to him.

Healing with the Chakras

When you sit with your animal, a good way to get the root of the problem is to run your hand over the animal's body, either on the fur or several inches above the body. See if you feel any areas that are warmer, colder, or murky feeling, compared to the rest of the body. These are generally good indicators of a disruption in the animal's energy field, and the best spots to place your hands and focus your loving attention.

Certain areas or illnesses may pertain to particular chakras, whose healing colors and properties you can further use to heal your animal.

4-legged animal chakra points are located in similar location between species. 2-leggeds also share similar points. So a dog's points are in the same location as a horse or a tiger, and a bird's is in a similar location to a human's or a kangaroo's.

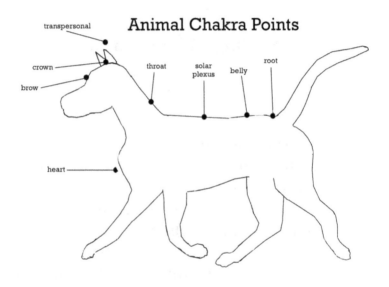

Root Chakra – The first chakra governs sex drive, reproductive organs, the legs and primal instincts. It is associated with the colors red, brown and black.

Belly Chakra – The second chakra rules digestion and issues relating to family and self-confidence. It is associated with the color orange.

Solar Plexus Chakra – The third chakra, associated with the color yellow, is concerned with the diaphragm, solar plexus and issues of safety, protection, and one's place in society.

Heart Chakra – The fourth chakra governs the heart, chest, and issues relating to forgiveness, love, stress and anger. It works with the colors green and pink.

Throat Chakra – The fifth chakra monitors the mouth, throat and respiratory system, as well as issues relating to voicing thoughts, speaking out. This chakra is often a turquoise or clear blue color.

Brow Chakra – The sixth chakra oversees the eyes, nasal passages and issues of the conscious mind. This chakra is associated with the colors purple and indigo.

Crown Chakra – The seventh chakra pertains to the head and issues of the soul, and is generally seen as white, gold or silver.

Higher Self Chakra – The eight chakra connects the crown chakra with the higher self and the astral body. Allows one to access their higher purpose in life. This is often gold or a radiant white comprised of all colors.

To learn more about chakras and associated illnesses, two books written for humans but whose basic message holds true for all species are: *Anatomy of the Spirit*, by Carolyn Myss and *Heal Your Body*, by Louise Hay.

For more information about energy healing for animals, see the Earth Lodge Guide *Energy Healing for Animals and Their Owners*, by Sandra Cointreau.

Bibliography

Ausubel, K. *When Healing Becomes a Crime: The Amazing Story of the Hoxsey Cancer Clinics and the Return of Alternative Therapies*. Rochester, VT: Healing Arts Press, 2000.

Beston, H. *Herbs and the Earth: An Evocative Excursion into the Lore & Legend of Our Common Herbs*. David R. Godine, 1935.

Brennan, B. *Hands of Light : A Guide to Healing Through the Human Energy Field*, NY: Bantam, 1988.

Broken Bear Squier, T. *Herbal Folk Medicine: an A to Z guide*. Owl Books, Henry Holt & Co., 1997.

Carper, J. *Miracle Cures: Dramatic New Scientific Discoveries Revealing the Healing Powers of Herbs, Vitamins, and Other*

Natural Remedies. HarperCollins Publishers, 1997.

Castleman, M. *Nature's Cures*. Rodale Press, 1996.

Cichoke Ph.D, A. *Secrets of Native American Herbal Remedies*. Avery, 2001.

Culpepper, N. *Culpepper's Complete Herbal*. W. London: Foulsham & Co.

Dobelis, I.N., Editor. *Magic and Medicine of Plants*. Pleasantville, NY: The Reader's Digest Assoc, 1990.

Duke, J.A. & Foster, S. *Peterson Field Guides: Eastern/Central Medicinal Plants*, Boston: Houghton Mifflin Company, 1990.

Emery, C. *The Encyclopedia of Country Living*.

Firebrace, P. & Hill, S. *Acupuncture: How It Works, How It Cures*. Keats Publishing, 1994.

Fischer-Rizzi, S. *The Complete Aromatherapy Handbook: Essential Oils for Radiant Health*. Sterling, 1991.

Fleischman, Dr. G. *Acupuncture: Everything You Ever Wanted to Know*. Station Hill Openings, 1998.

Grandin, Dr. T. *Animals in Translation: Using the Mysteries of Autism to Decode Animal Behavior*. Harvest Books, 2006.

Gray, P. *The Organic Horse: The Natural Management of Horses Explained*. David & Charles, 2001.

Green, M. & Keville, K. *Aromatherapy: A Complete Guide to the Healing Art*. The Crossing Press, 1995.

Griffin Ph.D., J. *Mother Nature's Herbal*. Llewellyn Publications, 1997.

Harris, B.C. *Better Health with Culinary Herbs*. Barre Publishers, 1971.

Heinerman, Dr. J. *Natural Pet Cures: Dog & Cat Care the Natural Way*. Prentice Hall Press, 1998.

Hofve DVM, J. *www.littlebigcat.com*

Hopman, E.E. *A Druid's Herbal*. Destiny Books, 1995.

Hutchens, A. *Indian Herbology of North America*, Boston: Shambhala, 1973.

Hylton, W.H. & Kowalchik, C. *Rodale's Illustrated Encyclopedia of Herbs*:Rodale Press, 1987.

Integrative Medical Arts Group. *Hepatotoxic Herbs*. IBISmedical.com, 1998 –2000.

Kavasch, E.B. & K. Baar. *American Indian Healing Arts: Herbs, Rituals, and Remedies For Every Season of Life*. NY: Bantam. 1999.

Kavasch, E.B. *The Medicine Wheel Garden: Creating Sacred Space for Healing, Celebration, and Tranquility*. NY:Bantam Books, 2002.

Kavasch, E.B. *Native Harvests: American Indian Wild Foods Guide*. Expanded & Revised Edition. NY: Dover Publications, 2005.

Kavasch, E.B. *Native Harvests: American Indian Wild Foods & Recipes*. Expanded. Washington, CT: Institute for American Indian Studies, 1998.

Kidd, J.S. & Kidd, R.A. *Mother Nature's*

Pharmacy: Potent Medicines from Plants. Facts On File, Inc., 1998.

Maclean, D. *To Hear the Angels Sing,* 1980.

Macrae, J. *Therapeutic Touch: A Practical Guide*, NY: Alfred A. Knopf, 1987.

Maleskey, G. *Nature's Medicines.* Rodale Press, 1999.

Manniche, L. *An Ancient Egyptian Herbal.* British Museum Press, 1989.

McCulloch M, See C, Shu XJ, et al. Astragalus-based Chinese herbs and platinum-based chemotherapy for advanced non-small-cell lung cancer: meta-analysis of randomized trials. *Journal of Clinical Oncology.* 2006; 24:419-430.

Medical Economics. *PDR (Physician's Desk Reference) for Herbal Medicine.* Thomson Healthcare, 1998.

A Medieval Herbal. Chronicle Books, 1994.

Meeus, C. *Secrets of Shiatsu.* Dorling Kindersley, 2000.

Gladstarr, R. & Hirsch, P. *Planting the Future: Saving Our Medicinal Herbs.* Healing Arts Press, 2000.

Motz, Julie. *Hands of Life: From the Operating Room to Your Home, an Energy Healer Reveals the Secrets of Using Your Body's Own Energy Medicine.* NY: Bantam, 1998.

Mulholland BSc BVMS Farrier, J. "Laminitis"

National Center for Complimentary and Alternative Medicines: National Institutes of Health. http://nccam.nih.gov

National Genetic Resources Program (NGRP). More than 80,000 plants in the data base. http://www.ars.grin.gov/

Null Ph.D., G. *The Complete Encyclopedia of Natural Healing.*

Peterson, L. & Peterson, R. *A Field Guide to Edible Wild Plants.* Houghton Mifflin, 1999.

Rand, W.L. *Reiki: The Healing Touch.* Vision Publications, 1998.

Restoring the Earth: Visionary Solutions from

the Bioneers. Tiburon, CA:HJKramer, Inc, 1997.

Richardson, M.A., et al. "Flor*Essence herbal tonic use in North America: a profile of general consumers and cancer patients." *HerbalGram* 2000(50):40-46.

Roberts, Monty. *The Man Who Listens to Horses: The Story of a Real-Life Horse Whisperer.* NY: Random House; 1996.

Rose, J. *Herbs & Things.* The Berkeley Publishing Group, 1972.

Self, Hilary Page. *A Modern Horse Herbal.* Buckingham, UK: Kenilworth Press. 1996.

Schiller, C. & Schiller D. *500 Formulas for Aromatherapy: Mixing Essential Oils for Every Use.* Sterling Publishing, 1994.

Schnaubelt, K. *Medical Aromatherapy.* Frog Ltd., 1999.

Schoen, A.& Wynn, S.G.. *Complementary and Alternative Veterinary Medicine: Principles and practice.* NY: Mosby/Times Mirror. 1998.

Schoen, A. & Proctor, P. *Love, Miracles, and*

Animal Healing: A Heartwarming look at the spiritual bond between animals and humans. NY: A Fireside Book/ Simon & Schuster, Inc. 1996.

Schoenbart L.Ac., B. *Chinese Healing Secrets.* Publications International, 1997.

Shamsa, F., Ahamadiani, A., & Khosrokhavar, R. *Antihisminic and anticholinergic activity of barberry fruit in the guinea-pig ileum.* Journal of Ethnopharmacology, 1999;64:161–166.

Sigerist, H.E. *A History of Medicine.* Oxford University Press, 1951.

Stein, D. *Essential Reiki: A Complete Guide to an Ancient Healing Art.* The Crossing Press, 1995.

Stein, D. *Natural Healing for Dogs & Cats.* The Crossing Press, 1993.

Stojakowska A., Kadziaan B. & Kisiel W. Antimicrobial activity of 10-isobutyryloxy-8,9-epoxythymol isobutyrate. Fitoterapia, 2005: Volume 76, Issues 7-8, Pages 687-690.

"The Ancient Herbal Tea that Became a Modern Cancer Tonic," in *The Doctors' Prescription for Healthy Living. Vol. 7 (8):* "Complementary Cancer Therapeutics." 2003.

Tierra, L. *The Herbs of Life: Health & Healing Using Western & Chinese Techniques*. The Crossing Press, 1992.

Wang, S.Y. and Zheng, W. "Antioxidant Activity and Phenolic Compounds in Selected Herbs". Journal of Agricultural and Food Chemistry, Vol. 49, No. 11: November, 2001.

Worwood, V. *The Complete Book of Essential Oils and Aromatherapy*. New World Library, 1991.

Yesilada E. & Kupeli E. *Berberis crataegina DC. root exhibits potent anti-inflammatory, analgesic and febrifuge effects in mice and rats*. Journal of Ethnopharmacology, 2002 Feb;79(2):237-48.

Von Muggenthaler, E. *The Felid Purr: A Healing Mechanism*. Fauna Communications Research Institute, 2001.

Resources & Supplies

ABCHomeopathy
www.abchomeopathy.com

Alaskan Essences
www.alaskanessences.com

Ameriherb
www.herbalcom.com

Aura Cacia Essential Oils
www.frontiercoop.com

Bulk Apothecary
www.bulkapothecary.com

Earth Lodge Essences
www.earthlodgeessences.com

Enchanted Realms
www.enchantedrealmz.com

Green Hope Farm Flower Essences
www.greenhopeessences.com

About the Author

Maya Cointreau is a certified Reiki master in the Usui tradition, herbalism and a shamanic lightworker with over 20 years of experience. Herbalism is a continuing passion, and she is constantly reading new science reviews, books and journals to keep up with the "discoveries," as science sets about proving what folk herbalists have always known: Herbs work.

At Earth Lodge, Maya has spent the last 15 years formulating herbal remedies for animals, creating new flower essences, and providing hands-on healing therapies for people and animals alike. You can visit Earth Lodge on the internet at www.earthlodgebooks.com.

"Authors like cats because they are such quiet, lovable, wise creatures, and cats like authors for the same reasons." ~ Robertson Davies

CPSIA information can be obtained
at www.ICGtesting.com
Printed in the USA
LVHW081327181121
703732LV00011B/200